Falling Awake

MEDITATION IS NOT WHAT YOU THINK: Mindfulness and Why It Is So Important
THE HEALING POWER OF MINDFULNESS: A New Way of Being
MINDFULNESS FOR ALL: The Wisdom to Transform the World

MINDFULNESS:
Diverse Perspectives on Its Meaning, Origins, and Applications
(editor, with J. Mark G. Williams)

MINDFULNESS FOR BEGINNERS:
Reclaiming the Present Moment—and Your Life

THE MIND'S OWN PHYSICIAN:
A Scientific Dialogue with the Dalai Lama on the Healing Power of Meditation
(editor, with Richard J. Davidson)

LETTING EVERYTHING BECOME YOUR TEACHER:
100 Lessons in Mindfulness

ARRIVING AT YOUR OWN DOOR:
108 Lessons in Mindfulness

THE MINDFUL WAY THROUGH DEPRESSION:
Freeing Yourself from Chronic Unhappiness
(with Mark Williams, John Teasdale, and Zindel Segal)

COMING TO OUR SENSES:
Healing Ourselves and the World Through Mindfulness

EVERYDAY BLESSINGS:
The Inner Work of Mindful Parenting
(with Myla Kabat-Zinn)

WHEREVER YOU GO, THERE YOU ARE:
Mindfulness Meditation in Everyday Life

FULL CATASTROPHE LIVING:
Using the Wisdom of Your Body and Mind to Face Stress, Pain, and Illness

FALLING AWAKE

How to Practice Mindfulness in Everyday Life

JON KABAT-ZINN

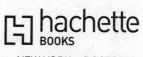

NEW YORK   BOSTON

Hachette Books
Hachette Book Group
1290 Avenue of the Americas
New York, NY 10104
hachettebooks.com
twitter.com/hachettebooks

Originally published in hardcover as part of *Coming to Our Senses* by Hyperion in January 2005.

First Edition: August 2018

Credits and permissions appear beginning on p. 171 and constitute a continuation of the copyright page.

Hachette Books is a division of Hachette Book Group, Inc.
The Hachette Books name and logo are trademarks of Hachette Book Group, Inc.

The publisher is not responsible for websites (or their content) that are not owned by the publisher.

The Hachette Speakers Bureau provides a wide range of authors for speaking events. To find out more, go to www.hachettespeakersbureau.com or call (866) 376-6591.

Library of Congress Control Number: 2018934793

ISBNs: 978-0-316-41175-2 (trade paperback), 978-0-316-52197-0 (ebook)

Printed in the United States of America

LSC-C

10 9 8 7 6 5 4 3 2 1

for Myla
for Stella, Asa, and Toby
for Will and Teresa
for Naushon
for Serena
for the memory of Sally and Elvin
and Howie and Roz

for all those who care

for what is possible

for what is so

for wisdom

for clarity

for kindness

for love

CONTENTS

What do we mean when we talk about "cultivating mindfulness"?

There is no question that mindfulness is one of the hardest things in the world for us humans to tap into consistently (even though it is not a "thing"), and even though we can taste it and recognize that experience of tasting in an instant, in any instant.

The invitation is always the same: to stop for a moment—just one moment—and *drop* into wakefulness. That is all. Stop and drop: meaning, drop in to your experience of experiencing, and for even the briefest of moments, simply holding it in awareness as it is—in no time, or to put it differently, in this timeless moment we call now, the only moment we actually ever have.

Luckily, if we miss this moment because we are distracted by one thing or another, caught up in thinking or in our emotions, or with the busyness of what always seems to need getting done, there is always the next moment to begin again, to stop and drop into wakefulness in this moment of now.

It seems so simple. And it is.

But it is not easy.

In fact, looked at one way, a moment of mindfulness, with no agenda whatsoever other than to be aware, is just about the hardest thing in the world for us humans to come to. And it is even harder for us to string *two* moments of mindfulness together.

And yet, paradoxically, mindfulness doesn't involve *doing* anything at all. In fact, it is a non-doing, a radical non-doing. And right inside any moment of non-doing lies peace, insight, creativity, and new possibilities in the face of old habits of mind and old habits of living. Right in that or any moment of non-doing, you are already OK, already perfect, in the sense of perfectly who and what you are. And therefore, right in that moment you are already at home in a profound way, far beyond who you think you are and the ideas and opinions that may so shape and sometimes severely limit your view of the larger whole. Not to mention your own possibilities for experiencing that wholeness and benefiting from it. And most interesting of all is the realization that there is no "that moment" at some other time, except in thought. In actuality, there is only *this* moment for dropping in.

None of this means that you won't get things done. In fact, when your doing comes out of being, when it is truly a *non-doing*, it is a far better doing and far more creative and even effortless than when we are striving to get things done without an ongoing awareness moment by moment. When our doing comes out of being, it becomes an integral and intimate part of a love affair with awareness itself, and with our ability to inhabit that space in our own mind and heart and to share it with others who are also engaged in that way of being as well—potentially all of us.

And none of this means, as is described in considerable detail in all four books in this series, that what you are experiencing has to always be pleasant—either during formal meditation practice or in the unfolding of your life. It won't be. And it can't be. The only reason mindfulness is of any value is that it is profoundly and completely up to the challenge of relating wisely to any experience—whether it is pleasant, unpleasant, or neutral, wanted or unwanted, even horrific or unthinkable. Mindfulness is capable of meeting and embracing suffering head-on, if and when it is suffering that is predominating at a particular moment or time in your life.

We don't learn much, if anything, about non-doing in school,* but most of us have experienced moments of radical non-doing as children. In fact, tons of them. Sometimes it comes as wonder. Sometimes it looks like play. Sometimes it emerges as concern for someone else, a moment of kindness.

Another way to put it is that mindfulness is all about *being*, as in "human being," and about life unfolding here and now, as it is, and embraced in awareness. Therefore, it takes virtually no effort because it is already happening. All it requires is learning to reside in your direct experiencing of this moment, whatever it is, without necessarily thinking that it is particularly "yours." After all, even "you" is just a thought construct when you put it under the microscope and examine it. If you do, you may discover that who you think you are is a very small and at least partially inaccurate account of who and what you actually are. In an instant, you can recognize how large the full dimensionality of your own being really is. You are already whole, already complete—as you are. And at the same time, you are part of a much larger whole, however you care to define it. And that larger whole, let's call it the world, sorely needs that fully embodied and more realized version of you.

Our wholeness manifests in everyday life as wakefulness, as pure awareness. Our awareness is an innate human capacity,

---

* That is, unless mindfulness has become part of the curriculum in your local school, which is happening more and more throughout the country and in different parts of the world.

one that we hardly ever pay attention to or appreciate or learn to inhabit. And ironically, it is already yours, conventionally speaking. You were born with it. So you don't need to acquire it, merely to familiarize yourself with this dimension of your own being. Your capacity for awareness is more "you" and more useful than virtually anything else about you, and that includes all your thoughts and opinions (important as it is to have thoughts and opinions, as long as we don't believe them and cling to them as the absolute truth).

And since the paradox is that all of us are already who we are in our fullness, this means that in the cultivation of mindfulness, there is literally no place to go, nothing to do, and no special experience that you are missing or are supposed to have. The fact that you are able to experience anything at all is already extremely special. Ironically however, the truth of that is hardly ever recognized, as we quest for that special something that always seems to somehow elude or frustrate our desiring—perhaps that perfect meditative moment in your own fantasy of what meditation should produce if you were "doing it" correctly.

There is nothing to acquire because you are missing nothing and lack for nothing, despite what your habitual patterns of thinking and wanting might be telling you in any given moment. You are already whole, already complete, already alive in this moment, already beautiful just as you are. So no "improvements" are either necessary or possible. This is it!

The only thing we are missing is *recognizing* the actuality of life unfolding in this moment—in the form of "you," in the form of "me"—in every dimension of that unfolding in the timeless present we call now, and *realizing* it, allowing it to be apprehended and thus made real in its fullness. There are no words for this because words are merely, for all their power and beauty when strung together skillfully, elements of thinking *about* things and thus once removed from direct apprehension. At this point, we enter the domain of pure poetry, where we attempt to use words to go beyond words, to convey what is not possible to say in a prose sentence. At this point, we are tapping into what one colleague* tellingly calls *implicational holistic meaning*—much more akin to directly feeling something and knowing it in one's bones, in one's heart, way beneath the words and concepts we may apply to the experience later. Perhaps in the end, it is this capacity that makes us human rather than automatons. And it is precisely here that we intersect with the domain of embodied mindfulness practice.

The mystery of awareness is that it is truly beyond words. It is intrinsic to our being. We all already have it and we always have. It is closer than close. Yet paradoxically, I have already used an awful lot of words to direct you toward apprehending something that is already yours, and already you—who you truly are just by virtue of being human. I hope that my pointing to it in words resonates with you and *in* you at a deeply intuitive level, way beyond words and stories.

This book and the others in this series are full of words, thousands of them. And yet, none of them are anything but pointers, sight lines for you to look along, feel along, sense along as you stop and drop, stop and drop, stop and drop in, moment by moment. Into what? Whatever is most at hand, most relevant, most salient to you in the moment. Into the actuality of now, of things as they are.

Simple? Yes! Can you do it? Of course you can! Does it involve

---

* See J. D. Teasdale and M. Chaskalson "How Does Mindfulness Transform Suffering II: The Transformation of *Dukkha*." In: *Mindfulness; Diverse Perspectives on Its Meaning, Origins, and Applications*, J.M.G. Williams and J. Kabat-Zinn (Eds) (Routledge, Milton Park, UK, 2013) pp. 103-124.

doing? Not really. Yes and no. It only looks like it involves doing. What it really involves is falling awake. And that, as we have seen, is a love affair with what is, and with what might be possible in the next moment if you are willing to show up fully in this one without any expectations or attachments to an outcome.

If you think of meditation as a doing, you might as well not pursue it—unless, that is, you also recognize that there is method in the apparent madness or nonsensicality of non-doing. In the ancient Chinese Chan [Zen] tradition, this is sometimes spoken of as *the method of no method*. This is where recognizing the unity of the instrumental (doing, getting things done) and the non-instrumental (non-doing) approaches covered in Book 1 comes in. Our intrinsic wakefulness can't be hyped. It can't be sold. It can't be corrupted. It can only be pointed to and realized. And the only way to realize it is to get out of your own way for a moment and simply stop and drop in, stop and drop in, stop and drop in.

One convenient way to do that is by attending to experience via your senses.

So we can experiment: Is it possible for us to come to our senses right in this moment? Can we hear only what is here to be heard? Can we see only what is here to be seen? Can we feel only what is here to be felt? Is it possible for us to wake up to the actuality of this moment of now and to what we might call our truest nature—what lies *underneath* all our thinking, our concepts, perspectives, world models, religious teachings, philosophies, scholarship, etc.? None of that is essential to the process of falling awake—although, paradoxically, any and all of it might be beautifully relevant as long as you aren't attached to it. The key is non-identification with anything as "I," "me," or "mine," because we actually have no idea (or only ideas) about who and what those personal pronouns actually refer to. Thus, just asking "Who am I?" and then stopping and dropping into awareness, into not-knowing, underneath thinking, is the beginning and the end of all meditative practices. Stopping and dropping in. When? Whenever you remember. How about now? And now? And now? Nothing needs to change. You don't have to do anything. Only remember.

*

As the world becomes more and more complex, and our days are filled with endless things to do and then cross off our to-do-lists, or moments when we are called to not just stand there but to do something, it is easy for us to become more and more entrained into narratives in our heads about what is going on and who we are in relationship to it all—about where we are going, or hope we are, or fear we might not be—and, in the process, lose touch with much of the beauty and wonder of being alive in the first place.

We construct identities, agendas, and futures for ourselves in our own minds, and then lose ourselves in those constructs, in our models of reality, and in our thoughts, which, even if they are true, are only true to a degree, definitely not entirely true, and usually not true enough. By that point, we are probably too busy, too caught up in the momentum of all the doing in our lives to remember that we could also be awake. We so easily default to an automatic pilot mode—descending into the familiar ruts in our thinking and our emotional life, getting caught up in going from agenda item to agenda item, and becoming more and more addicted to all the ways we have to distract ourselves through our devices and our so-called "infinite connectivity"—that we lose sight of what is right in front of us and of what is called for now, and now, and now.

The cultivation of mindfulness, both formally and informally, can pop that bubble right in the moment it arises, or as soon as we recognize what is happening. It can uncover and help us recover hidden dimensions of ourselves that we will need going forward more than ever if we are to be true to our own humanity and its full flourishing in the form of you. None of us wants to have "I should have spent more time working" or "I wish I had been more distracted" on our gravestone, but many of us act that way in how we allocate our energies and in the sum total of our missed moments. Mindfulness can be a counterbalance to all of that without forcing any of it to stop. It is only *we* who have to stop, and only for this timeless moment.

Since this book is about how to practice mindfulness in everyday life, let's be clear about it...there is nothing other than everyday life.

Nothing is excluded from everyday life, including all the thoughts and emotions we might be having in any moment, no matter what is happening. In essence, if something is arising, whatever it is, it is taking place within the domain of our life. And so it becomes part of the "curriculum," you might say, of mindfulness in that moment. (And if it is recurring, it becomes part of the curriculum in many many moments—because sometimes the curriculum doesn't let go of *us*.) In the end, *all* our moments can be part of the cultivation of mindfulness, not just the times during the day that we carve out for formal meditation practice. Life itself becomes the curriculum. Life itself becomes the meditation practice.

Herein lies the very essence of the cultivation of mindfulness and of coming to our senses both literally and metaphorically. If we only have this one life to live, are we going to sleepwalk through it, lost in our thoughts and narratives and our emotions? Or are we going to find ways to wake up to the fullness of this moment and of what it might portend if only we were more in touch with and accepting of it and of ourselves in the face of anything and everything that can arise during a single moment or over the course of a day? This book invites you (and I should also say "us," since I am no exception, and we are working together on this exploration and adventure, along with millions of others who choose to orient their lives in this way) to practice falling awake, moment by moment throughout the day. And also to practice it more formally at specific times, by setting aside stretches of clock time that are dedicated solely to being, with no agenda for doing or accomplishing anything (including even secret agendas for getting better at meditating!). The fullness of your experience in any moment is already complete, so there is no improving on it. The challenge is always, can we be here with it, for it, *in* it until we realize that whatever is unfolding in a particular moment is the curriculum of that moment? And thus realizing, as the old *New Yorker* cartoon of two monastics in conversation after a period of formal meditation suggests, "Nothing happens next. This is it."

In these pages, from one end of the book to the other, we will be cultivating embodied wakefulness. Each chapter is really a different door into the same room: the room of your own awareness. Each doorway, and each of our senses of course, has its own unique and quite wonderful features. What unifies the practice though is that the room we are entering is the space of our own awareness, no matter which doorway we choose to enter through. We literally or metaphorically take our seat and ground ourselves in the practice without editing or judging whatever is arising in experience from moment to moment. As best we can, we do so without getting caught up in asking ourselves whether we are having a "good" meditative experience, or whether what we are experiencing is what we are "supposed" to be experiencing. If you are having it and you are aware of it, whatever you are experiencing is perfect for that moment—and perfectly what it is.

The real question is: "How are you going to be in relationship to whatever is unfolding in any particular moment that always turns out to be this one?" In other words, can you hold what you are experiencing in awareness without judging it in any way or creating a narrative that you wind up believing *about* your experience—pleasant, unpleasant, or neutral? The willingness to rest in awareness with whatever your experience of the moment may be (wanted, unwanted, or barely noticed; pleasant, unpleasant, or neither) invites *a new way of being in relationship to experience altogether*, including just how judgmental we are! It carries with it a new possibility of inhabiting a space of freedom far bigger than your likes and dislikes and your favorite perspectives on how the world works or doesn't. And thus, for even the briefest of moments, it invites you to simply be who and what you already are—beyond your own name, your "story of me," beyond thought altogether, or we might say, *underneath* your thinking.

What you will find is no secret, but at the same time it is a hidden gold mine. It is your own awareness embracing clear seeing, and thus greater wisdom. It is equanimity, and thus an unwavering stability of mind and heart, nurtured by deep caring and concern. It is an intrinsic love affair with life beyond our too-small narratives of who we are and how the world is. As we saw in *Meditation Is Not What You Think*, apprehending who and what we actually are in our fullness and how and what the world actually is in its fullness is a radical act of love and sanity. And this opens us up to the possibility of acting at least a bit more wisely in this world, and thereby experiencing the healing and transformation and liberation that come with those actions, moment by moment and day by day.

So the suggestion is to throw yourself into the formal and informal practices offered here as if there were no tomorrow, as if your entire life hung in the balance. Because in very real and important ways, your life *does* hang in the balance. And so does the full potential of your presence and effectiveness in the world, in your family, in whatever you chose to do, and in your very body and the way you carry yourself (and your body carries you) in the world.

This engagement takes a certain discipline and resolve. If you possibly can, it means to every day, whether you feel like it or not, both metaphorically and literally, get your rear end on a meditation cushion or a chair (or bed) and keep it there for longer than you feel comfortable doing so. It means putting out the welcome mat for the inevitable discomfort, impatience, boredom, mind-wandering, and plague of everything else that will arise. It means inviting them all to become your teachers and to help you shape how you choose to be in relationship with it all—the wanted and the unwanted, the pleasant and the unpleasant, the easy and the difficult. Herein lies not torture (although sometimes it can feel that way) but freedom—the freedom of not being caught in and possibly imprisoned by your own liking and disliking or endless narratives, none of which are true enough. In this mirror, the mind wakes up. It comes to know itself, to befriend itself and all experience. And in the process, you, whoever you are, come into being that knowing. In the process, you will know far better both how to be, and when doing is called for, what to do.

Have fun. And stay in touch. Especially with yourself. And know that you are not alone in cultivating wakefulness in all these various ways. We are all in it together, stretching the envelope, giving ourselves over to the practice formally and informally as best we can, and seeing/apprehending what emerges, and what is so for now.

Jon Kabat-Zinn
Berkeley, CA
February 20, 2018

PART 1

The Sensory World

Your One Wild and Precious Life

Who made the world?
Who made the swan, and the black bear?
Who made the grasshopper?
This grasshopper, I mean—
the one who has flung herself out of the grass,
the one who is eating sugar out of my hand,
who is moving her jaws back and forth instead of up and down—
who is gazing around with her enormous and complicated eyes.
Now she lifts her pale forearms and thoroughly washes her face.
Now she snaps her wings open, and floats away.
I don't know exactly what a prayer is.
I do know how to pay attention, how to fall down
into the grass, how to kneel down in the grass,
how to be idle and blessed, how to stroll through the fields,
which is what I have been doing all day.
Tell me, what else should I have done?
Doesn't everything die at last, and too soon?
Tell me, what is it you plan to do
with your one wild and precious life?

MARY OLIVER, "The Summer Day"

The Mystery of the Senses and the Spell of the Sensuous

Every object, well contemplated, opens a new organ of perception in us.

Johann Wolfgang von Goethe, eighteenth-century German polymath

What is capable of seeing, hearing, moving, acting has to be your original mind.

Chinul, twelfth-century Korean Zen Master

Our senses and what they give rise to are, when well-contemplated, mind-boggling in every respect. We tend to take them sorely for granted and underappreciate their scope and depth, if we appreciate them at all. Our senses undergird our capacity to recruit and develop an astonishing array of intelligences for decoding experience and situating ourselves in the phenomenological world. Being in touch with our senses—considerably more than five, as modern neuroscience is showing—and the worlds they open us to inwardly and outwardly is the essence of mindfulness and meditative awareness. Attending to them provides myriad opportunities for realizing wakefulness, wisdom, and interconnectedness in our everyday lives.

Under special circumstances, our senses can become extraordinarily refined. It is said that aboriginal hunters in Australia, living in the outback, could see the larger moons of Jupiter with the naked eye, so keen was their hunting vision. When one sense is lost at birth or before the age of two, it seems the other senses may take on qualities of acuity far beyond what we usually think possible. This has been shown in various studies, even with sighted people deprived of sight for relatively short periods of time, from days to hours. They show, in Oliver Sachs's words, "a striking enhancement of tactile-spatial sensitivity."

By simply being in a room with people, Helen Keller could decipher using her sense of smell "the work they are engaged in. The odors of the wood, iron, paint, and drugs cling to the garments of those who work in them... When a person passes quickly from one place to another, I get a scent impression of where he has been—the kitchen, the garden, or the sickroom."

The various isolated senses (we tend to think of them as separate and non-intersecting functions) all subtend different aspects of the world for us, and facilitate the construction and knowing of the world from raw sensory impressions and our relationship to them. Each sense has its own unique constellation of properties, out of which we build not only our "picture" of the world "out there" but out of which we build meaning and our moment-to-moment capacity to situate ourselves within it.

We can learn a great deal about ourselves and what we take entirely for granted from the reported experiences of those who do not have one or more of the sense capacities most of us share, whether it was that way from birth or as a result of later loss. And we can ponder what the experience of such profound loss (at least it feels that way to us) would be, and gain insight from those who have found ways to live fully within such constraints. Thus, we might come more to appreciate the gifts of those senses available to us in this moment, and of our virtually limitless potential to put them to use in the service of our own hopefully always-growing awareness of the inner and outer landscapes of our lives. For what we know we know only through the full spectrum of the senses, coupled with that capacity of mind that we might call knowing itself, its own kind of sensory and integrative function.

Helen Keller writes:

I am just as deaf as I am blind. The problems of deafness are deeper and more complex than those of blindness. Deafness is a much worse misfortune. For it means the loss of the most vital stimulus—the sound of the voice that brings language, sets thoughts astir and keeps us in the intellectual company of man...If I could live again I should do much more than I have for the deaf. I have found deafness to be a much greater handicap than blindness.

The poet David Wright describes the experience of his deafness as seldom being devoid of a sense of sound:

Suppose it is a calm day, absolutely still, not a twig or leaf stirring. To me it will seem quiet as a tomb though hedgerows are full of noisy but invisible birds. Then comes a breath of air, enough to unsettle a leaf; I will see and hear that movement like an exclamation. The illusory soundlessness has been interrupted. I see, as if I heard, a visionary noise of wind in a disturbance of foliage...I have sometimes to make a deliberate effort to remember I am not "hearing" anything, because there is nothing to hear. Such non-sounds include the flight and movement of birds, even fish swimming in clear water or the tank of an aquarium. I take it that the flight of most birds, at least at a distance, must be silent...Yet it *appears* audible, each species creating a different "eye-music" from the nonchalant melancholy of seagulls to the staccato of flitting tits...

John Hull, who lost his sight completely in his late forties, gradually experienced a loss of all visual imagery and memory and a descent into what he calls "deep blindness." According to Sachs, writing about the senses in the *New Yorker*, being a "whole-body seer" (Hull's term for characterizing his state of deep blindness) involved shifting his attention, his center of gravity, to the other senses, and, Sachs notes, Hull "writes again and again of how these have assumed a new richness and power. Thus he speaks of how the sound of the rain, never before accorded much attention, can now delineate a whole landscape for him, for its sound on the garden path is different from its sound as it drums on the lawn, or on the bushes in his garden, or on the fence dividing it from the road."

"Rain has a way of bringing out the contours of everything; it throws a colored blanket over previously invisible things; instead of an intermittent and thus fragmented world, the steadily falling rain creates continuity of acoustic experience...presents the fullness of an entire situation all at once...gives a sense of perspective and of the actual relationships of one part of the world with another."

Sachs's phrase "never before accorded much attention" is telling here. Necessity fosters and furthers such an according of attention in those who are missing one or more of the senses. But we do not have to experience the loss of our sight or hearing, or any other sensorium, to accord attention to it. It is the invitation of mindfulness to meet our sense impressions at the point of contact (see *Meditation Is Not What You Think*, "The Origin of Shoes"), and to know and linger in the knowing of these worlds in their fullness, rather than in their diminution through our ignoring or habitually dulling of both the sense gates themselves and the mind that encounters them and accords them and ourselves meaning.

Just as we can learn and be astonished by the capabilities of those who have suffered the loss of one or more sense and made extraordinary accommodations and adjustments in both body and mind to fashion a full life, so we can learn from purposefully according some attention to the natural world, which beckons to us and offers itself to us through all our senses simultaneously, a world in which our very senses were fashioned and honed, and in which we have been seamlessly embedded from the beginning.

Although we tend not to notice it, we perceive across all our senses simultaneously in any and every moment. Even in Wright's description and Hull's there are cross-references to the lost sense. Wright has to remind himself that he is not hearing what he is seeing, for it "appears *audible*" to him, manifests as "eye-music." And Hull, who has no visual experience, nevertheless speaks of "a colored blanket" thrown "over previously invisible things," suggesting that they are indeed made "visible" through his careful hearing.

The senses overlap and blend together, and cross-pollinate. This experience is called *synesthesia*. We are not fragmented at the level of our being. We never were. Our senses, blending together, shape our knowing of the world, and our participation in it from moment to moment. That we do not recognize this is merely a measure of our alienation from our own feeling body and from the natural world.

David Abram, whose book *The Spell of the Sensuous* looks

deeply into the crosscurrents of phenomenology and the natural world as it is sensed and known by all the creatures that inhabit it, including ourselves when we dwell in the wild, shares with us the rich dimensionality of the sensory matrix that gave birth to us and nurtured us for hundreds of thousands of years.

The raven's loud, guttural cry, as it swerves overhead, is not circumscribed within a strictly audible field—it echoes *through* the visible, immediately animating the visible landscape with the reckless style or mood proper to that jet black shape. My various senses, diverging as they do from a single, coherent body, coherently *converge*, as well in the perceived thing, just as the separate perspectives of my two eyes converge upon the raven and convene there into a single focus. My senses connect up with each other in the things I perceive, or rather each perceived thing gathers my senses together in a coherent way, and it is this that enables me to experience the thing itself as a center of forces, as another nexus of experience, as an Other.

Hence, just as we have described perception as a dynamic participation between my body and things, so we now discern, within the act of perception, a participation between the various sensory systems of the body itself. Indeed, these events are not separable, for the intertwining of my body with the things it perceives is effected only through the interweaving of my senses, and vice versa. The relative divergence of my bodily senses (eyes in the front of the head, ears toward the back, etc.) and their curious bifurcation (not one but *two* eyes, one on each side, and similarly two ears, two nostrils, etc.) indicates that this body is a form destined to the world; it ensures that my body is a sort of open circuit that completes itself only in things, in others, in the encompassing earth.

Immersed and embedded in the natural world, we only know it through our senses, and we are known through the senses of other beings, including beings that are not human but who sense us all the same in their own ways, whether it be a mosquito looking for lunch or birds announcing our arrival in a forest glen. We are part of this landscape, grew up in it, and are still the possessors of all its gifts, although compared to our hunter-and-gatherer ancestors, ours may have atrophied somewhat from lack of use. But the spell of the sensuous, in Abram's enticing and entrancing phrase, is no further than the sound of the rain taken in, or the feel of the air on the skin, or the warmth of the sun on our backs, or the look in your dog's eye when you come near. Can we feel it? Can we know it? Can we be embraced by it? And when might that be? When? When? When? When? When?

SEEING

We do a lot of looking: we look through lenses, telescopes, television tubes... Our looking is perfected every day—but we see less and less. Never has it been more urgent to speak of seeing... we are on-lookers, spectators... "subjects" we are, that look at "objects." Quickly we stick labels on all that is, labels that stick once—and for all. By these labels we recognize everything but no longer see anything.

FREDERICK FRANCK, *The Zen of Seeing*

There is a field near my house that, seen from a certain angle, particularly delights my eye. I pass by the bottom of this field several times a day and in all seasons as I walk with our dog. Sometimes I am alone, sometimes with other people, sometimes even without the dog. It doesn't matter. The field is continually offering a curriculum of light and shadow, form and color to the passerby, evoking the challenge to sense and drink in in any and every way whatever is delivered to eyes, ears, nose, palate, and skin. Every day, every hour, every minute, with every passing cloud, in every weather, with every season, what is here to be seen is different, perpetually changing, morphing with the light and the heat and the season from one aspect to another, like the landscapes of mountains and gorges and the fields of haystacks that enticed Monet to paint from the same spot on multiple easels as the day unfolded, as the seasons turned, capturing the uncapturable light and its mysterious birthing of shape and texture, color, shadow, and form. The challenge for us is to see that such a display offered up by the world that we inhabit is in fact everywhere. Yet this particular field, resting as it does on the slope of a gentle and uneven hill, with two outcroppings of fieldstone adding to its unevenness, has a special catalytic effect on me, especially when seen from below. Gazing upon it, I am somehow changed, recalibrated, more finely tuned to both inner and outer landscapes.

It lies nestled on the hill, sloping up to the east between two other flat fields above and below that are conservation land and so grow wild, mostly with grass. To the north is the back of a faded red barn and beyond that, a cobblestone driveway and an old but well-kept New England farmhouse, white, segmented, obviously elongated over the years, stretching section by skillfully added section toward the oldest, nearest the road. Another conservation field on the same slope lies to the south, separated from the fenced-in one by a double row of tall oaks and chokecherries on either side of and over-arching a low rock wall no doubt dating to colonial times when the land was first cleared for planting and all the ancient dug-up, black-granite stones piled wide and massively along the edges.

The field that so captures my eye has a three-tier wooden fence around it with two hardly visible electric wires set off from each fence post by very visible yellow spacers, set there to contain the two young cows our farmer neighbor keeps there part of each year, his "babies." The fence describes a markedly irregular pentagon that for a long time I perceived as a rectangle. Then it took on the look of a trapezoid. Only with extended gazing did it finally reveal itself as actually five-sided. The western, lowermost side of the fence parallels the eastern one above it and these two are connected to the south as if they were the long facing sides of a rectangle, the shorter connecting side mounting straight up the hill, paralleling the double line of trees and the rock wall just to its south. Twenty feet or so to the north past the small cow shed built into the bottom western side, the fence cuts diagonally northeast up the hill for a ways. Then there is a gate where this sloping side meets the shortest, fifth side, that joins up with the top edge in a right angle. This configuration gives both field and fence an unstudied and unruly look that hugs the contours of the hill and fits perfectly within the sweep of this landscape. From the bottom right (southwest), my favorite vantage point, the whole of the field is visible except for the interior of the cow shed and what the shed obscures in my line of sight.

I love this particular field. For some mysterious reason, walking below it and unavoidably gazing upon it enlivens my seeing. All is suddenly more vivid in the world.

I sit in this moment in the shade gazing up on the hill from the southwest vantage. The sun hangs fairly high in the mid-morning sky on this 4th of July, soaking the field in intense light and heat. A narrow, continually expanding line of shade advances right to left from the southern edge, courtesy of the row of trees. The field is overgrown, the grass tall, dried to browns and golds, gone completely to seed. Droplets of white hang above it, dabbed there by an abundance of wild daisies the cows haven't got to cropping yet. White butterflies flutter here and there, and an occasional dragonfly, the large kind, patrolling low and fast over the grass through the languid air like the marvelous, improbable, Carboniferous creature that it is, with its two pairs of delicately laced, transparent, extremely versatile wings, on the wing in search of mosquitoes. Two scrub trees stand in the field by themselves in the southwest corner right in front of me, and a few bigger ones shade the shed from either side. Already there is a hot hazy feel to the day. The sky behind me is blue, mostly cloudless, yet in my field of vision, the sky above the field, fringed by the large, more distant trees beyond the upper field, is entirely white.

Walking back along the path below the field and farmhouse after sitting in the grass gazing at the field for some time, the expanses of red fescue to my left are somehow redder than when I came. Now I am seeing large splotches of purple here and there in the grass, what may be flowering wild peas, which I had barely noticed before. The yellow lilies abundantly populating cut-out circles at the edges of the large lawn are more yellow, their micro-motion—almost a bouncing in the light breeze—more apparent to my eye. I see far more dragonflies nearby than I had earlier, and notice how the swallows, which before I barely saw at all, are flitting and swooping in low over the tall grass, back and forth across the lawn to the ample dabbles and streaks of oranges and pinks, reds, blues, purples, and golds (the farmer loves his flowers), all defined by an overflowing magnificence of brilliant yellow cedum with its succulent greenery spilling along the expansive horizontal lines of a two-tiered rock wall garden that rises from the far edge of the huge lawn below the house.

When I come to the road I turn right, uphill, for veritably it is all the same hill, toward my house, knowing that later this afternoon, the field and the walk I will take along the same trajectory will be entirely different, and that difference will make me different, will require me to be different, meaning present afresh for what will be offered up to the senses in whatever moment I arrive. And it is always so, summer or winter, spring or fall, yesterday or today, in rain and gloom and snow, at night under the stars...I am always arriving. It is always already here, just as it is, always the same field, but never the same.

In walking these paths, there is less and less separation between me and the view when I give myself over to attending, when I allow myself to come to and live within my senses. Subject (seer) and object (what is seen) unite in the moment of seeing. Otherwise it is not seeing. One moment I am separate from a conventional scene as described to myself in my head. The next moment, there is no scene, no description, only being here, only seeing, only drinking in through eyes and other senses so pure they already know how to drink in whatever is presented, without any direction at all, without any narrative at all, without any thought. In such moments, there is only walking, only standing, only sitting, or for that matter, only lying in the field, only feeling the air.

Of all the senses, it is vision, the domain of the eyes, that dominates in language and metaphor. We speak of our "view" of the world, and of ourselves; of gaining "insight" and "perspective." We exhort each other to "look" and then to "see," which is as different from looking as hearing is from listening, or smelling is from sniffing. Seeing is apprehending, taking hold, drinking in, cognizing relationships, including their emotional texture, perceiving what is actually here. Carl Jung observed that "We should not pretend to understand the world only by the intellect; we apprehend it just as much through feeling." Marcel Proust put it this way:

The true journey of discovery consists not in seeking new landscapes but in having fresh eyes.

We see what we want to see, not what is actually before our eyes. We look but we may not apprehend or comprehend. We all have our blind spots and our blindnesses. Yet we can, if motivated, tune our seeing just as we can tune an instrument, thereby increasing its sensitivity, its range, its clarity, its empathy. The goal would be to see things more as they actually are rather than how we would like them to be or fear them to be, or only registering what we are socially conditioned to see or feel. If Jung was correct, we apprehend with our feelings, yes, but then we had best be intimate with them and know them for what they are or they will provide only distorted lenses for any real seeing or real knowing.

One way or another, as it does with the other senses, our own mind often obscures our capacity to see clearly. For this reason, if we wish to experience life fully, and take hold of it fully, we will need to train ourselves to see through or behind the appearances of things. We will need to cultivate intimacy with the stream of our own thinking, which colors everything in the sensory domain, if we are to perceive the interior and exterior landscapes, including events and occurrences, to the degree that they can be known, in their actuality, as they truly are.

*

Starting here, what do you want to remember?
How sunlight creeps along a shining floor?
What scent of old wood hovers, what softened
sound from outside fills the air?

Will you ever bring a better gift for the world
than the breathing respect that you carry

wherever you go right now? Are you waiting
for time to show you some better thoughts?

When you turn around, starting here, lift this
new glimpse that you found; carry into evening
all that you want from this day. This interval you spent
reading or hearing this, keep it for life—

What can anyone give you greater than now,
starting here, right in this room, when you turn around?

WILLIAM STAFFORD,
"You Reading This, Be Ready"

BEING SEEN

My wife, Myla, and I sometimes do an exercise with people who come to our mindful parenting workshops that involves remembering back to a moment in your childhood when you felt completely seen and accepted for who you were by an adult, not necessarily a parent, and dwelling in the feeling tone and images conjured up by the memory.

Alternatively, if no such memories of being seen in childhood arise when invited, you are invited to notice, if they arise instead, moments in which you felt unseen, disregarded, not at all accepted for who you were by an adult in your life.

It is amazing how quickly and how vividly moments of being seen and fully accepted arise for us in memory when invited in in the safety of such a gathering. Stories emerge of quiet moments digging in the dirt as a child with one's grandmother, or of a parent simply holding one's hand while gazing into a river, or of someone dropping an egg on the floor on purpose after you had done so by accident, just so you wouldn't feel alone or ashamed. These memories arise spontaneously, often without having ever been consciously recalled before. They have been here with us our whole life, never forgotten, for we are not likely to forget, even as children, moments of feeling completely seen and accepted.

Most of the time such moments are without words. They often unfold in silence, in a parallel play of doing together and being together wordlessly. Perhaps there is merely the exchange of a glance or a gaze, a smile or a sense of being held or hugged or your hand taken and held. But you know in that moment that you are seen and known and felt, and nothing, nothing in the world, feels better, puts you more at ease and sets the world aright, puts you more at peace. Even if there is only one such memory in us, we carry it forever. We never forget it. It is in there. It is in here, because it meant so much, revealed so much, honored so much. It was more of a gift than we could consciously know. But intuitively, we knew. The body knew. The heart knew. And we knew non-conceptually. And in the knowing, we were moved, and are moved to this day by the memory.

It is also amazing how few such memories any of us have, and how many of us have no such memories. Instead, there may be recollections of moments in which we felt distinctly unseen, unaccepted, even shamed and ridiculed for being as we were.

The message from such an exercise for parents is, of course, that every moment with our children is an opportunity for us to see our children as they are and to accept them fully at any and every age. If such moments of being seen were so important for us as children that we have never forgotten them, even if they were extremely rare or singular, then why not be mindful of the healing power of such quiet presence as can come from seeing your children at least in some moments beyond your expectations for them, beyond your fears, and your judgments, and even your hopes. These moments can be fleeting, but if inhabited and embraced, they are deep nourishment, an oxygen line of lovingkindness straight into the heart of the other.

So our regard (from the French *regarder*, to look) is itself a worthy object of attention, to be held in awareness and the consequences of it seen, felt, and known. For it is not just seeing that is important. There is also its reciprocal, being seen. And if that is true for each of us, it is true for all of us, for any and every other.

Seeing and being seen complete a mysterious circuit of reciprocity, a reciprocity of presence that Thich Nhat Hanh calls "interbeing." That presence holds us and reassures us and lets us know that our inclination to be who we actually are and to show ourselves in our fullness is a healthy impulse, because who we actually are has been seen, recognized, and accepted, our core sovereignty-of-being acknowledged, embraced.

All this is part of the reciprocity of seeing when seeing is true seeing. When the veils of our ideas and opinions thin enough so we can see and know things as they are rather than staying stuck in how we desire them to be or not to be, our vision becomes benign, tranquil, peaceful, healing. And it is felt by others as such, instantly. It is felt, it is known, and it feels very very good.

It is not just children and other people who know when they are being looked at and can feel instantly the quality and intent of a gaze. Animals know it too, and sense how it is that we are seeing them, with what qualities of mind and heart, whether in fear or in gladness. And women, of course, know and have always known the ominous, depersonalizing, objectifying, sometimes predatory aggression of a certain male gaze unsoftened by caring and by an honoring of the sovereignty of the other.

Some ancient native traditions believe that the world feels our seeing, and sees us right back, even the trees and the bushes, even the rocks. And certainly, if you have ever spent a night alone in the rain forest or the woods, you will know that the quality of your seeing and of your being is felt and known by Abram's "more than human world." You will sense that you are definitely being seen and known for what you really are, if not exactly how you normally think of yourself, and that whether you are comfortable with it or not, you are an intimate part of this one animate and sensuous world.

*

Only the garden was always marvelous. No one had cared for it for a very long time, and it had gone back to seed and wildflowers. Its beauty was in a subtlety only careful watching could perceive.

GIOIA TIMPANELLI, *Sometimes the Soul*

*

There they were, dignified, invisible,
Moving without pressure, over the dead leaves,
In the autumn heat, through the vibrant air,
And the bird called, in response to
The unheard music hidden in the shrubbery,
And the unseen eyebeam crossed, for the roses
Had the look of flowers that are looked at.

T. S. ELIOT, "Burnt Norton," *Four Quartets*

HEARING

Old pond,
frog jumps in—
splash.

BASHO (1644–1694)

Heavy early-morning mid-November rain is hitting the roof in the darkness above my head. Every moment, there is the sound of it. Can I hear it…beyond my thoughts about the rain, even for one moment? Can I "receive" these sounds as they are, with no concepts whatsoever, including the concept of sound? I notice that hearing happens effortlessly. I don't have to do anything. There is nothing to do. In fact, in order to really hear, "I" have to get out of the way. My "I" is extra. There is no need for a "me" that is hearing, or looking out for the sounds, that is, listening. In fact, I notice, that is precisely where all the thinking is spouting from, from expectations, from ideas about my experience.

I experiment: Can I simply let sound come and meet the "ear consciousness" that arises in the bare experience of hearing, as is already happening in any and every moment? Is it actually possible to get out of my own way and just let there be hearing, to let the sounds come to the ear, be in the ear, in the air, in a moment, without any embellishment, without any trying? Just hearing what is here to be heard, since the sounds are already rapping at the gateway of the ears. Being with hearing in the stillness of open attending. Drip, drip, drip, gurgle, gurgle, gurgle, swirl, swirl, swirl... the air filled with sound. The body bathed in sound. In utter stillness, there is only the rain on the roof, whipped sometimes by the wind into sheets spattering on the windows, pure sound in the ears, filling the room.

In this moment, somewhere, far in the background, there is the knowing that I am sitting here, that rain is falling, but the experience "before thinking," behind any thoughts that do secrete themselves, is one of pure sound, just hearing, no longer a separate hearer and what is being heard. There is only hearing, hearing, hearing...And in the hearing, the knowing of sound, beyond words like "rain," beyond concepts like "me" and "hearing." The knowing rests in the hearing. For now, they are one.

This rain is so forceful this morning, so compelling, so absorbing, that attention sustains itself effortlessly. The experiencing of sound has in this moment trumped the conceptual mind. This is not always or even usually the case. It is so easy to be carried into thinking. It is so easy to distract myself, to be carried so far away from the ears that I do not even hear the rain anymore, no matter how forceful, even though the body and the ears are still just as bathed in its sounds as the moment before, when there was only "just this..."

So, an elemental challenge of mindfulness is to rest in the awareness of hearing, hearing only what is here, moment by moment by moment, sounds arising, passing, silence inside and underneath sounds, beyond interpreting the momentary experience as either pleasant or unpleasant or neutral, beyond all identifiers and judgments, beyond all thoughts about anything, just this giving myself over to sitting, hearing, breathing, knowing....

In the hearing, there is momentary freedom from any "me" hearing, and from what is heard, from both a knower and what is known. Nothing is missing. A moment of original mind, empty, knowing, vast. For a brief moment perhaps, we have actually come to, arrived at, our senses. Can we abide here for a time? Can we live here? What would we lose? What might be gained? Recovered? When are sounds and the spaces between sounds not present for us? When are sights not present to us? Are we here for them? Can we be here with them? Can we be the knowing, rest in the knowing, act out of the knowing, fully present with what already is? What is the feeling tone of such a moment?

Trying is not the answer. We do not have to try to hear. But the mind is devious. Can we know it? Can we know it?

Even in Kyoto—
hearing the cuckoo's cry—
I long for Kyoto.

BASHO

*

Be a person here. Stand by the river, invoke
the owls. Invoke winter, then spring.
Let any season that wants to come here to make its own
call. After that sound goes away, wait.

A slow bubble rises through the earth
and begins to include sky, stars, all space,

even the outracing, expanding thought.
Come back and hear the little sound again.

Suddenly this dream you are having matches
everyone's dream, and the result is the world.
If a different call came there wouldn't be any
world, or you, or the river, or the owls calling.

How you stand here is important. How you
listen for the next things to happen. How you breathe.

WILLIAM STAFFORD, "Being a Person"

SOUNDSCAPE

It is 6:42 a.m. in late June. Through open windows, I am bathing in the sounds of birds I do not know, trills and whistles, warbles and clicks, calls and responses, short and long, some soon recognized in repeats, others not so easily distinguished again, all modulated, syncopated, melodiously and chaotically spilling into the air, filling the world with song under song over song, within song, after song. It goes on and on in a clamor, moment by moment, ever new, ever exuberant, a cornucopia of sound spilling out everywhere.

There is also the not-too-distant and unmistakably growing hum of traffic on a not insignificant artery flowing intently deep into the body of the metropolis toward the heart of the city from the northwestern periphery, and pouring out in the other direction under similar pressure. The occasional roar of a semi accelerating is discernible but for the most part, the impatient tire whirs and insistent engine purrs merge into one sound stream announcing that the world of human purpose and industry is waking from its slumbers along with the birds.

Delicious soundscape, punctuated at times by the fluttering of leaves on the gigantic Norway maple behind me, so close to the house, and by sighing from the boughs of the hemlocks in front of me caressed by intermittent gusts of gentle wind, all coupled with, just now, the conversational voices of dog walkers passing by in the unpaved street under those hemlocks. Now a siren sound is contributed, distinct, brief, not repeated, and now and again a bang from something heavy being dropped off a truck on the farm below the hill. There are also beeps from something big backing up somewhere. This soundscape is always present. It is always the same and always different as the minutes and hours flit by. And always, in each moment, there are the birds' songs and occasional screeches.

I cease thinking any thoughts about sources and give myself over to hearing. It is very much a bathing in sound, a sensuous luxuriating in pure sound and the spaces between them, in layer upon layer of sounds. Now they are simply what they are, no longer identified, no longer listened for in a straining, reaching sort of way. I simply sit here moment by moment, receiving whatever is arising in the soundscape, not even inviting it to come to my ears, since it is always coming anyway, if mostly not really heard or known because the mind is elsewhere, preoccupied with something, anything at all, which can always include thinking about the origins of the sounds I am hearing or preferring some to others, having opinions instead of just hearing.

In this giving myself over to the hearing, pure and simple, in these moments there is only the hearing. The soundscape is everything. It is no longer in the world. It is the world. Or, more accurately, there is no world anymore. And no me listening, and no sounds "out there." There are no birds, no trucks, no airplanes and sirens and ladders being put up. There is only sound and the spaces between sounds. There is only the hearing in this all-of-a-sudden timeless moment of now, even as it flows into the next timeless moment of now. And in the hearing, there is also the immediate knowing of sound as it is heard in its arising, in its brief or sustained lingering, in its passing away. Not the knowing that comes with thinking but a deeper knowing, a more intuitive knowing, a knowing that is somehow before the words and concepts that clothe our knowings, something underneath thinking, more fundamental... the co-arising with sound of the knowing of sound as sound, as just what it is, before it gets dressed up by the thinking mind and evaluated by our naming, by our liking and disliking of things, by our judging mind. It is something like a mirror for sound, this knowing, simply reflecting what comes before it, without opinion or attitude, open, empty, and therefore capable of containing anything that presents itself.

In this moment, the immersion is so complete that there is no longer any immersion. Sound is everywhere, the knowing is everywhere, within the envelope of the body and without, for there is no longer a boundary of any sort. There is only sound, only hearing, only silent knowing within an infinite soundscape, only this, only just this....

That is not to say that thoughts do not arise. They do. It is rather to say that their presence no longer colors the hearing or interferes with it. It is almost as if the thoughts themselves have become sounds and are heard and known along with everything else, in their arising and in their passing. They no longer distract or disturb, for in being known, they tend to melt away, no longer proliferating endlessly. The knowing is skylike, airlike. Like space, it is everywhere, boundless. It is nothing other than awareness itself. Pure. Utterly simple. It is also utterly mysterious for it is not something that I am creating but rather a quality not separate from being alive that sometimes emerges, like a shy animal come to sun itself on a log in a forest clearing. It lingers if I am quiet and don't make sudden movements within the space of the mind.

The clock before me now shows 8:33. In these hours an infinite number of moments have gone by—and yet no time has passed. I feel anointed, blessed by this bathing, by this immersion in a soundscape that knows no beginning and no ending, by this miracle that is hearing, that is wakefulness, that is knowing. I wonder if there is any moment in which this "just this" is not available to me. What does it take to hear what is always already here to be heard, punctuated and buoyed as it always is by an even greater underlying silence?

I do notice, later on, that if I am not careful, meaning grounded in awareness as the day unfolds, within no time I might be hearing nothing for hours on end other than the roaring noise of the thought stream in my own head—no matter what is presenting itself to the ears.

*

Meditating with a group of environmental activists on a rocky beach on Windfall Island, at the mouth of Tebenkof Bay in the Tongass Wilderness in southeast Alaska, just off Chatham Strait and across from the snowcapped peaks of Baranov Island, none of us can but take note of how the humpback whales contribute hugely to the ambient soundscape in this pristine wilderness air as they come and go with the tides day and night between the bay and the strait. We hear the whoosh of their out-breath, long, deep, sonorous, and so basic, so ancient, it is as if we are immersed in breath sounds that have been going on uninterrupted for millions of years in the same place, which of course, they have. If we are sensitive enough, we occasionally hear the in-breaths as well, just before they dip back under. With eyes open, we can see as well as hear their out-breaths, even from quite a distance, as the white vapor geyser bursts forth high into the air with every surfacing. We feel they somehow know we are here on the beach, sitting, our eyes closed for the most part. For a time we are immersed in a world that is probably little different from the way it was five or fifteen thousand years ago or more, a vast and primordial silence, ebbing with sounds. Bald eagles cry out, ravens squawk, smaller birds on the water and in the air all contribute their various calls and cries, the waves lap at the shore, the wind blows through old-growth Sitka spruce and western hemlock temperate rain forest that has known the force of the brutal winters but never the clear-cut saw. We sit here, opening to this world, to this soundscape, to its ancient memories. Or are they certainties?

*

Our dog knows that the soundscape includes what is not heard every bit as much as what is. If she hears the screen door open and close, but does not hear it slam shut and click, she knows she can escape the house. She just knows. This is merely an example of how not hearing in the soundscape is full of significant information, if we are tuned in enough to detect the absence of sounds, and changes in patterns of sound and silence. Music may tickle our auditory nerves, as Taj Mahal used to sing it, but the soundscape isn't just sound, it is the entire universe of sounds and silences, shared by our hearing when we are willing to give ourselves over entirely to just being, nothing more, just being with hearing.

There is a sound like a garbage truck outside as I sit here. It is not garbage day. Perhaps it is a street sweeper, says my mind, seeking some way to identify it. But it is not going away. Maybe they are drilling. It sounds like a truck going up a steep incline forever, not getting nearer or farther away. Perhaps they are doing some work up the street. I can sit here and think endless thoughts about it, where it is coming from, how much I wish it weren't here, why it is happening so early in the morning. Maybe I should get up and investigate, see where it is coming from, what is making that noise.

To what end? Right now, I am sitting here. I can choose to be disturbed or not. But that choice seems difficult and remote, an exercise of willpower, a way of resisting what is already so, already here, this sound. I watch the disturbance and non-disturbance oscillate back and forth.

Behind this play of my mind is pure sound. Hearing the sound and not knowing "what" it is are both knowing. In this moment, can I simply rest in that knowing, the knowing that doesn't know and doesn't need to know, and is content because these sounds are already here in this moment? Things are already just like this right now. Can they be accepted as they are because anything else is going to lead to disliking, to frustration, to disturbance, to greater distraction?

The mind secretes a thought...perhaps I could accept it better if I knew what it was, who was making it, how long it was likely to go on.

Awareness also knows that thought as a thought as it is emerging. It sees the thinking mind groping, grasping, desperate now for some kind of explanation, for reassurance, for a coordinate system within which acceptance might reside, having managed to turn what were just sounds into noise, a magical if unnecessary alchemy. Awareness also sees these thoughts, the annoyance, the struggling, and the grasping as extra, as equally unnecessary. They are impediments to tranquility, impediments ironically far greater than the sound itself. There is tranquility in the hearing and in the knowing underneath the sound. I let go into it. The sound stops momentarily, then resumes. No hindrance arises.

All of a sudden, the mind experiences a spasm of discomfort. It insists on finding out. Somehow, awareness and my larger purpose evaporate. The spasm of desiring to identify the source gets the body up to look out the window.

A big truck is going by. It is a noise, but not *the* noise. What has getting up and looking done for me? Nothing.

I resume sitting, and settle in to hearing. The urge to find out grows enormous the longer the sound goes on. I continue sitting, and disappear into it. After a while, the sounds move off into the distance and birdsongs reemerge. Thinking comes up with something else, even now that things are more quiet. That is seen. A smile is spreading across my face. Breath moving in and out. Sitting here, just sitting here sitting...a spaciousness no longer tainted by thoughts of sounds or of silence. Awareness. There are no longer any interruptions. The mind no longer interrupts itself. For now, there is only just this. Just this.

The sound comes back. The smile widens, lingers, dissolves.

AIRSCAPE

Imagine yourself under water, still fully able to breathe.

Now try moving.

Move just one arm and hand, slowly at first. Can you "feel" how the "water" streams around the arm, between the fingers, across the back of the hand and all around? As I do it now, I feel a fluidity in the movement itself, as if my arm and hand suddenly have a new life to them. They seem drawn to go on their own wherever they can, to flow and undulate anywhere and everywhere, to experiment spontaneously with greater freedom of motion. These slow, inherently elegant movements seem to become more fluid merely by imagining and thereby sensing that they are in a fluid.

If you are doing it now, can you feel how graceful your moving has already become? And how effortless? Linger in this feeling as long as you like while continuing to move. And if you like, gradually let the rest of your body join in. Let yourself become a strand of kelp waving rhythmically in a bed of waving kelp in the ocean near where sea meets land. You might try standing up if you are sitting, and let your whole body, arms, legs, torso, and head, move however it likes, feeling the flowing currents around the body as it is drawn into responding in whatever ways it chooses to the fluid within which it is immersed.

Actually, we do live at the bottom of an ocean—an ocean of air. Letting go of the water image, you might play with seeing if you can actually *feel* this ocean of air with your skin as you move your arms and hands as slowly as before, feeling the streaming of the air through and around your fingers and hands, bathing in the sensations you are experiencing, whatever they are. As you settle more and more into your body and bring more and more awareness to the body as a whole, allowing it to move on its own, in its own way, perhaps noticing how the felt sense of the body moving can turn amazingly, instantly, into the essence of tai chi—flowing movement within stillness, within an ocean of awareness, an ocean of air.

Now allow yourself to come to stillness and sense the air with your whole body. Rather than searching for a particular feeling, let it emerge on its own, as if you were listening with your skin for the air to speak. You do not have to reach out or try to do or feel anything. After all, the air is already all around you and inside you, touching you.

Without trying, sensing how you are already embedded in this fluid, how the ocean of air caresses your skin, envelops you, embraces you, even when it is hardly moving in a room, even when it is utterly still. Feel how you are mysteriously drawn to draw it into your body over and over again through your nose or mouth, how this happens without your trying, without any forcing, without volition even. Feel how it is received by the baskets that are your lungs, and reflect for a moment on how the oxygen molecules, unimaginably tiny, are magically snared out of the air that has diffused from the alveoli in your lungs into the bloodstream by the correspondingly enormous but still unimaginably tiny hemoglobin molecules packed into now—in the binding with oxygen—bright red blood cells that do only the job of transporting that air essence with every contraction of the left ventricle of your heart to all the trillions of cells that make up the infinitely complex universe of your body, all of which would soon die without this essential sustenance. Such a reflection might give occasion to pause for a moment, allowing you to metaphorically catch your breath and consciously situate yourself in the airscape.

Myself, I am currently having an on-again, off-again love affair with the air. When I remember, the love affair is on. When I forget, it is off again until the air itself re-minds me, and re-bodies me.

Not that it is hard to love the air. In summer, light morning breezes flow over bare shoulders as I sit in stillness, breathing with eyes closed, or open. I feel the air around the body with my skin and lo, the skin is enlivened. I bathe in the sometime gusts and subtler currents in the room, drink in the humidity and the freshness, and I am of a sudden more awake. The dankness of a sometimes heavy evening speaks in its own tongue to skin and nose, every bit as much as do the excitations of a sea breeze square in my face, the balm of a midwinter thaw, and the bite of a January wind that freezes skin anywhere it is exposed.

It wasn't always so. For most of my life, the air was just the air, not really noticed at all and appreciated even less. Slowly the realization has crept up on me that it is indeed just air, but what a gift. What a sensuous gift, this invitation to feel what is already offered to us, to experience that we are being perpetually embraced and nourished, at all times both touched by and touching the spirit of Ariel, the very air itself. We are breathing and being breathed. We are living in air, like Chagall figures, and living on it and off it too.

When I relate to the air with a degree of affection, intimacy, and constancy, that is, with increasing mindfulness, it is hard not to notice that the airscape is continually in flux. One moment it is moving, the next moment it is still. It beckons me, awakens me, keeps me on my toes when I feel it in this way. Now it is warm. I look and feel again, and it is cool. Its various personas are met in different hours, in its different seasons. The sweet back-to-school coolness, full of memories, the bracing chill of winter, more memories, and the occasional warm day with a feeling all its own for not being summer but pretending, while snow and ice are all around, melting, and giving the air its own unique signature of feels and smells.

The air, the air, the air. Once you begin paying attention to it, loving the air, you can easily understand why it was elevated and revered as a primordial element by ancient civilizations. The air! The air! As I look out at the stand of hemlocks, they are swaying, playing at their tai chi. I feel the same air that is moving them moving now across my back and shoulders and neck. In this, we are united, touched by the very same wave, each moved and moving in our own ways, and also, amazingly, joined in an exchange that is larger than us both, in which all life, plant and animal, is participating in every moment around the entire planet, a giving and receiving between these large living kingdoms on a cosmic scale, a recycling and revitalizing of the air that also recycles and revitalizes us.

And this dynamic exchange, wonder of wonders, maintains this thin and strangely vulnerable invisible blanket of atmosphere that wraps and hugs our round home within the unthinkable vastness of the vacuum we call space, a vacuum of almost emptiness, almost nothing.

And that, from our point of view as living creatures, is

everything...because without the invisible air, we are soon nothing again ourselves.

> *Hast thou, which are but air, a touch, a feeling*
> *Of their afflictions?*

> W. SHAKESPEARE, *The Tempest*

Touchscape

It is not just the air that touches us, although its touch is constant. Our body touches every chair it sits on, every piece of floor or ground it stands on, every surface it lies on, every piece of clothing in contact with the skin, every tool our hands wield, every thing we attempt to grasp, lift, propel, receive, or deliver. And perhaps most importantly, we touch each other in myriad ways, sometimes automatic, sometimes perfunctory, sometimes sensuous, sometimes romantic, sometimes loving, sometimes aggressive, sometimes unfeeling, sometimes with anger. Depending on how we are touched, we can feel loved, accepted, and valued, or ignored, disrespected, assaulted. We touch through handshakes, a hand on another's shoulder, an arm around another, through pats, hugs, lifts, embraces, kisses, caresses, dances, massages, and, usually in games, where such touch is regulated by different sets of rules than our normal social code, through colliding, tackling, checking, grappling, even kicking and punching. And there are times when, not in games, we might be either touched or touching another in ways that are unkind, even menacing, or worse. Of course, increasingly there are laws regulating that kind of touch in society for the protection of our basic rights of safety and bodily sovereignty as individuals.

But however we touch and whatever we touch, inanimate or animate, plant, animal or human being, stranger, client, colleague, friend, child, parent, lover, we can touch either mindfully or mindlessly. And in any and every moment, we have a chance to know directly, through awareness, how we ourselves are being touched, and how we are feeling and what we are sensing from moment to moment as a consequence of both how we are touching and how we are being touched. This is the landscape of touch, the *touchscape*, if you will, the sensory field of ever-reciprocal direct somatic contact between ourselves and the world, which we can feel, whether superficial or deep, across any and every square inch of our bodies.

As I sit here cross-legged in this moment writing at my desk on the floor, I am aware of the sensations coming from my butt in contact with my meditation cushion (*zafu*), and from the outside lengths of my lower legs, stretching from knees to ankles and upturned feet, draped one in front of the other, resting on the fabric-enclosed cotton batting (*zabuton*) that cushions them from the floor. I am also aware of the touch sensations coming from the upper surfaces of my feet, which are also in contact with this padding. These are the only parts of my body at present in contact with what is beneath me, holding me up, even as gravity is continually pulling every part of the body toward the floor, completely balanced by the repose of the posture itself.

The dominant sensation at the moment is one of heaviness in the lower part of the buttocks extending just a bit into the upper thighs in back, where they are absorbing the pressure of the upper body pushing down into the well-stuffed zafu. The pelvis is tilted forward and the lumbar spine as a consequence curves in lordosis toward the abdomen so that the greatest pressure is on the bones lying beneath the gluteus maximi. There is a sense of contraction in the left knee more than the right, as the left leg, foot, and heel are closer to the perineum than the right leg, which lies beyond the left one in contact with the zabuton below it. The feeling of contraction gives a sense of the knee being somewhat congested in this moment. There are sensations of tingling and pulsing, almost throbbing, much more in this knee than in the other one. There is also the softness of the padding against the outer edges of the lower legs and the tops of the feet. I notice that some of the sensations in the legs and buttocks are from the contact with what my lower body is sitting on in this posture, but others, like the sensations in the knee, extend beyond this physical contact and include sensations that are simply associated with the body's awareness of itself and where all the various regions of the body are in relationship to each other and in relationship to the space it is occupying. This is part of the sensory experience of *proprioception*, from the Latin, *proprius*, meaning "one's own."

The rest of my body is touching only the air surrounding it, except for the contact of the heels of my hands with the laptop's hand rest, and the palm-side ends of my fingers pressing into the keys as I type at this close-to-the-floor table that serves as a desk when sitting in this fashion. Sensations in the heels of the hands include warmth (the laptop is giving off heat), the smoothness and the hardness of the surface they are lying on, and their own intrinsic heaviness. The heels of the hands, supporting the weight of the arms, feel anchored and weighty. The fingers, flexed in the customary position on the keyboard, feel light, energetic, and pulsing.

Of course, touch is not segregated from the other senses, so I am also aware in this moment of the *soundscape* bathing me by way of the air that bathes my skin and enters my lungs with every contraction of my diaphragm as I sit here. And I am touched by it, but in a different way than the direct somatosensory contact of the touchscape. It feels somewhat less tangible, more disembodied, until I realize that it is my whole body that is absorbing the sounds and not just my ears, that as I pay careful attention, the physical vibrations of the sounds are being felt in some cases right down to my bones.

I am also simultaneously aware of what is continually presenting itself to the eyes, what we could call the *sightscape*, the screen upon which these words are appearing—thirty years ago, in the era of electric typewriters, such an experience would truly have been considered science fiction—and beyond the screen, the room, and the early-morning sunlight through windows to my right illuminating just a few vertical surfaces, the back of the desk chair, a bit of the desk, a red loose-leaf book stuffed vertically next to the printer, the sun's own calligraphy—reflected shadows of a few leaves from the giant Norway maple outside—magically appearing on the vertical support for the shelving above the printer. I look again after a few minutes have passed and it is all different. The light on the desk gone. The shadow calligraphy is cast from a slightly different angle. The leaves and stems are now more defined, and flatter.

Ashley Montague, in his classic book *Touch: The Human Significance of the Skin*, observed that the word "touch" has the distinction of the longest entry in the *Oxford English Dictionary*. That means that it is longer even than the entry for the word "love." And, if we stop and think about it, it may not strike us as all that surprising. For where would love be without touch? Touch is so basic to life. (In high school biology class, when we looked at, poked, and probed cells and small animals under a microscope, this property was coldly and clinically referred to as "irritability.") We are embedded in the world and know it through all the senses, but the most basic one, the least specialized, the most global, has got to be touch, which transpires across the membrane of skin that contains us, defines our body, and differentiates its interior milieu from the outer, the world beyond its bounds. Before we were born, we all grew into our body and our being within the living environment of another being and her body, bounded within other membranes where we were held apart and yet somehow not apart as well, not quite two yet, not even separate bodies—containment and touch at their most basic. We know all this, yet somehow often forget or downplay the utter miracle and lived mystery of it. We have all participated in it from one side, and mothers from both.

We are nurtured through touch, nurturing touch, loving touch, loving containment, holding, before we are born and after. While latched on and nursing, babies usually feel around for the other nipple and hold on to it, touching and in touch with one through the lips and tongue, with the other through tiny perfect fingers, completing circuits of love and continual nurturing, nourishing connection, a sustenance well beyond the milk itself. When carried, babies are continually held and therefore touched, in contact with the larger bodies of their parents and caretakers. And when they sleep with their parents in their bed, the physical contact continues while sleeping, wrapped in the same warm and loving cocoon.

Metaphorically speaking, we can be out of touch, lose touch, be touched (as in the head), and feel touched (as in when our hearts are moved). We can not touch our food, put the touch on someone for money, feel a touch of envy or sadness, add a touch of paprika, have a touch of the flu, let the candlelight provide just the right touch, be told not to touch anything, touch off an uproar, touch upon something in conversation, touch up the scratches on our car, add finishing touches to the flower arrangements, and touch base with someone.

The sense of touch is actually, from a neurological point of view, a number of different senses all subsumed under the same word. Sensing the pressure of contact is one. Sensing the temperature of contact is another. Sensing contact that is so intense it causes us pain is yet another, as is sensing a caress so loving it gives us pleasure.

Another dimension of the sense of touch involves our ability to sense the body inwardly, to know, for instance, where your hands are without moving them or looking at them, or what the carriage of the body is in any moment. As we have already noted, this sensory capacity we all have is called *proprioception*, the sense of knowing where the body is spatially, orienting within the field of the body and sensing its movements and intentions.* Proprioception is so basic that we almost never accord it any status in awareness. It is taken completely for granted. But as we shall see in *The Healing Power of Mindfulness*, Part 1, loss of proprioception through sensory nerve damage is utterly catastrophic. One no longer knows or feels that one is, so to speak, a resident of the body, inhabiting a willing universe of potential intentional activity within the larger world. One's hands and legs are no longer one's own. They are foreign objects, with no value or utility. They cannot be moved in anything like the usual way. One's connection with them and with the whole of the body is severed. It is the ultimate being out of touch. Happily, this condition is extremely rare.

But being unaware of proprioception and being instrumentally out of touch with our own body is, sadly, extremely common. Luckily, in this case, there is an enormous amount we can do to

---

* Another term, *interoception*, is now used by neuroscientists to designate the sense of the physiological condition of the entire body and its continual regulation to maintain inner balance, or homeostasis—if you will, an "inward touching," giving rise to the condition of knowing how we feel.

recover this miraculous dimension of lived experience instantly, for it is never far away, always closer than close. We are only out of touch because we ignore what is already here. If we drop the ignoring, we come instantly to our senses because the senses are already and always delivering. That is their nature. We only need to awaken to them.

*

After rain after many days without rain,
it stays cool, private and cleansed, under the trees,
and the dampness there, married now to gravity,
falls branch to branch, leaf to leaf, down to the ground

where it will disappear—but not, of course, vanish
except to our eyes. The roots of the oaks will have their share,
and the white threads of the grasses, and the cushion of moss;
a few drops, round as pearls, will enter the mole's tunnel;

and soon so many small stones, buried for a thousand years,
will feel themselves being touched.

MARY OLIVER, "Lingering in Happiness"

In Touch with Your Skin

The skin is our biggest sensory organ. Someone calculated that in an adult it measures approximately twenty square feet of surface area if laid out flat, and weighs about nine pounds. We tend to label the skin as *the* organ of touch even though, as we've just seen, we are touched by the world through all our other, in some ways more specialized, sense organs as well.

But what the word "touch" most evokes for us is intimately tied to our skin. This is also true when we use the word "feel" in certain ways. For it is by way of the skin that what we think of as "physical" contact is made and felt, and it is here where the simultaneous bidirectional reciprocity of our contact with the world is most apparent. For we cannot touch something without being touched by it in the very same instant. We cannot be touched without touching. Walking barefoot, our feet kiss the earth with every step, and the earth kisses right back and we feel it. Of course, if we are "out of touch," we won't feel it even though the contact is undeniable. And as we know, the best way to be out of touch is for our mind to be distracted or preoccupied—caught up in ruminations, in the stream of thoughts and emotions, in our own self-involvements, as is so often the case, and therefore unavailable for direct experience in any moment. In this digital age, we are at risk for being permanently and perpetually distracted and self-distracting, requiring more presence of mind than ever before to stay in touch with what is most important—hence the increasing importance of mindfulness.

We also know that the skin is intimately tied to our emotions. If we let them, things can get "under our skin." We blush with embarrassment, are flushed with pride, turn white with fear, pale with grief, green with envy.

For all these reasons and many more, the skin is a magnificent object of meditative attention. Bringing awareness to our skin, we readily sense the air around the body, perhaps for the first time consciously. At first, it may be easier to feel the air touching the skin and our skin touching the air when there is a breeze blowing, but with cultivation, we can sense the air around the body at any time, even when the air is not moving, just by bringing awareness to the envelope of the body. The skin doesn't actually breathe. Still, it can be useful to sense or imagine it "breathing" across this membrane between our flesh and the rest of the biosphere by intentionally placing our mind on and in our skin. Our awareness can envelop the skin like a glove envelops our hand. Awareness soaks right into skin like water into a sponge. When we are mindful of the sensations in the skin, it can feel like our mind is inhabiting our skin. Mind and skin are not separate, except when the mind goes to sleep. You could even say, with some accuracy, that the skin is an aspect of the mind.

This is not as far-fetched as it may sound. As we shall see, there are a number of different maps of the body in the brain, one set of which is known as the somatosensory homunculus (see *The Healing Power of Mindfulness*, "Homunculus"). The regions of the somatosensory homunculus correspond to the surface features of the skin. But in the homunculus, the hands and feet and lips and tongue are huge compared to other locations on the skin. This is because of the high concentration of sensory nerve endings in these particular regions, refined sensing elements embedded throughout the thin membrane that is our skin and the tissue below it. So when you put your mind intentionally in your hands or feet, or in your lips, you will feel a vivid panoply of sensation coursing through the skin in these locations.

The skin is a sensory world unto itself. It is never devoid of sensation, even when it doesn't seem to be touching anything. For it is always touching something by virtue of being an interface. It has its own sensory tone at all times. It is always in touch. The question is, are we? Can we be in touch with our own skin?

You may also feel greater sensation in your hands and feet and lips because of the high enervation of motor neurons in these regions, especially in the hands. The sensory and motor functions go—dare I say it—hand in hand. Sensing your hands from inside, and right out through the skin, you will feel a beauty of form and function that is in no way secondary to any hands carved in marble by Michelangelo. We honor the artistry and aesthetic that "brings stone to life" in part because it reconnects us to our own intrinsic beauty, a beauty that transcends age and everything that has happened to us that may be writ large on and in the body in some way…it touches us. It reminds us that these are our miraculous hands that we so much don't know, that we so much take for granted, so much use mechanically, that we can ironically be so insensate to. When we perceive so palpably the life in the marble, we are brought back to life ourselves, resuscitated metaphorically and literally. It is another benefit of this unavoidable reciprocity embedded in sensing, in this case taking place at the interface where trafficking occurs between inner and outer worlds across the sturdy yet delicate surfaces of skin and fingers, our thumbs and our palms, the miracle of hands.

*

You are more beautiful than any one,
And yet your body had a flaw:
Your small hands were not beautiful,
And I am afraid that you will run
And paddle to the wrist
In that mysterious, always brimming lake
Where those that have obeyed the holy law
Paddle and are perfect. Leave unchanged
The hands that I have kissed,
For old sake's sake.

W. B. YEATS, "Broken Dreams"

SMELLSCAPE

Sitting on the porch of a Cape Cod house in mid-August, the salt air that I have known intimately since childhood carries intimations of the nearby sea to my nose. It has an unmistakably familiar fragrance, but almost indescribable in its complexity and its delicacy. Whenever I return to this place, I know I am getting close by the smells that mix the land and the sea into the air. It has moisture in it, this gently moving air this morning. I don't just feel it caressing my skin, I am smelling it now, especially as my attention narrows and sharpens to take it in. It carries a seaweed aroma, ever so faint, a wet sand aroma, an eel grass aroma, an aroma of all the plant and animal seashore life surrounding us on three sides in tidal pools and on the beaches. There is also the smell of damp dank earth from the nearby sassafras woods and wetlands, and occasional wafts of the hydrangeas in the flower garden, and from the uncut grass baking in the increasingly strong mid-morning sun. There is also the unmistakable earthiness of the shredded black mulch recently put down around the cedar trees, and also the faint smell of wet stucco being spread like nut butter onto the new house under construction next door.

But look what I have done. I cannot describe the smells themselves, nor the feel of this *smellscape*, except by analogy, or by naming objects and hoping they evoke something within you that might recollect places and times in which you had similar experiences and could remember the timbre of the fragrances. I cannot bottle the essence of this smellscape for you or for me. It is complex, infinitely rich, unique, and changing in every moment, all the while staying approximately the same. It cannot be contained, preserved, or transferred. I can name the possible sources but struggle to convey the actual experience. You would have to smell it yourself to know it, and even then, it would be hard for us to talk about and perhaps better if we didn't, richer and more sensory and sensible if we just remained silent in the experiencing of it rather than retreating, as we are so often apt to do when we have any kind of experience, into our heads and right into more or less mindless speech, a narrative that so easily kills the unspeakable richness of the silent sensing knowing sharing.

Fragrances offer us a world unto itself via our most delicately attuned sense. The nose can detect infinitesimal levels of aromatic compounds, a few parts per trillion in some cases. Smell is fundamentally a molecular sense, as is taste. Of course, smelling and tasting are closely related anatomically and functionally. When our nose is blocked up, it is hard for us to taste anything.

Molecules in the air are the source of all smell experiences other than those we generate solely through memory, when we somehow manage to excite the olfactory brain in just the right way to re-create a Proustian experience as vivid as the original. Even though our own olfactory prowess is meager compared to most animals, still it is the case that "nothing is more memorable than a smell." Our attraction or our aversion can be instant, reflexive, animal-like in nature when a scent is particularly pleasant or unpleasant. The long-evolved, some would say primitive, although there is little primitive about it, biological imperative of approach and avoidance always lurks at its most basic here in the world of smells, with us in its reflexive grip. Indeed, compounds known as pheromones link us to each other, help us find each other, and just as with other species of animals, participate in choreographing the social and sexual dances we engage in and the choices we make in deciding with whom to pass on our genes in new combinations to future generations. The search for chemical attractants that can be manufactured and marketed to the masses is now the Holy Grail for fragrance company laboratories. Small wonder.

With most smells, being neither too pleasant nor too unpleasant, well, we are likely to miss them altogether. Even with strong smells, the nose is soon saturated. A few moments of immersion and we are apt to smell nothing, not even noxious fumes. The nose is a fine instrument, but it tires quickly if overwhelmed. It's hard for us even to smell the food we are eating right through a meal.

Once again it is the air that mediates between source and detector, for the air delivers far more than sounds to our ears. Smells, scents, aromas, fragrances, stenches, and stinks travel its byways. Our dogs know them so much more vividly than we do, and often long before we do for those we can detect at all. Dogs inhabit a smellscape far richer than ours. Theirs is a predominantly smell-defined universe that provides them with huge amounts of relevant information, information about other dogs, people, and places, apparently whole histories and itineraries can be inferred. Apparently the olfactory epithelium in the nose (which is really where the business of smelling takes place) of a dog can have up to seventeen times the surface area of ours, and over one hundred times the concentration of smell receptors per square centimeter. The olfactory cortex of rats and shrews is a huge proportion of their entire cortex. In humans, that proportion is minuscule. Of course, shrews and dogs do not have the huge areas of cerebral cortex uncommitted to sensory and motor functions that allow for our far more elaborate cognitive and creative functioning.

Sometimes I think that the main purpose of walking my dog is to give her time to explore the wider world through her nose. Each spot she comes to is a public bulletin board of messages and notations announcing who and what have already passed this way, which other denizens of the neighborhood, canine and noncanine, are afoot. Many particular spots invite her, for reasons unknown to my senses, to roll on her back in the tall summer grass, her belly splayed open to the sky, head to one side; or, in winter, to respond to the scents and textures peculiar to deep snow recently fallen that resonate with her silver Siberian Husky genes. In such moments, she will stick her snout down into the snow and plow this way and that right over her eyes, taking in a world I am a stranger to. Without adequate time for smelling, I imagine her brain and her being, her husky essence are bereft, somehow not stoked in the ways they require daily, if not hourly or moment by moment, for her to be her full dog-self. She needs to be free to wander wherever her nose carries her, but this has its own problems in a human-dominated world. In any event, she is my meditation teacher in this, as in so many other ways. Really, she is walking me more than I am walking her. When I can remember this, I am in closer proximity to the more-than-human world. It helps me to step out of time, and out of my head.

People, countries, cities, villages, buildings and houses, landscapes, seascapes all have their signature aromas. A first whiff of New Delhi is never forgotten, and so it is for most places and seasons, except when we mask and sanitize them compulsively. Scents speak to us of many things, evoke many feelings, emotions that go way beyond nostalgia or mere memory. Scents and fragrances can plunge us into grief or ecstasy. And yet, and yet…they wake us up too, invite us to surrender entirely to the present, basking in the fragrance and the fragrances of now.

> *The wind one brilliant day, called*
> *to my soul with an odor of jasmine.*
>
> *"In return for the odor of my jasmine,*
> *I'd like all the odor of your roses..."*

> ANTONIO MACHADO
> *Translated by Robert Bly*

Perhaps it is not surprising that Machado feels an urgency in the demand for reciprocity between the odors in the wind and the fragrances within his own being. But were they ever separate?

TASTESCAPE

To give a sense of the *tastescape*, I thought I would eat one almond and try to describe the experience. I took it from the granola I made last week, so it was baked along with a lot of other things, including olive oil and maple syrup, lots of oats, sesame seeds, sunflower seeds, some cinnamon, and a little salt. As I put the almond in my mouth, I am struck by its size. It is quite large. I can feel the skin softening up and oops, all of sudden, there are two pieces in my mouth. I can feel the wrinkled skin on the one side, and the smooth surface of the seedling that it is, now split in two, on the other. I bite into them—perceive that they are surprisingly crunchy—and start chewing, slowly. The crunchiness rapidly turns to something with the consistency of cornmeal. It is amazing how the taste floods the mouth, peaks, and then trails off. It happened much faster than I thought it would. So, to zero in on the taste again, I put another in my mouth after swallowing what was left of the first one.

Slowly, mindfully chewing, chewing, tasting, tasting. Hmmmmm. Everything that is going on in the mouth is the domain of the tastescape, but what is it like in this instant?

It is definitely sweet, but in the subtlest of ways. If I had been blindfolded and just had it put in my mouth, I would know instantly from the taste that it was an almond. But would I know, from tasting, that it was an almond that has been marinated in other tastes? I am not sure. I couldn't really say I detect the cinnamon, but its presence probably explains in part why this almond tastes as it does. Same for the maple syrup and the oil and all the other ingredients. When all is said and done, here too, the taste itself is not readily describable—what does cinnamon taste like without using the word "cinnamon"?—but the experience of tasting is infinitely knowable if I am willing to linger with it silently. And perhaps I would know it as different if I were given an almond that had not been treated in this way, not roasted, not part of a granola made with tender loving care.

Last night at a local restaurant I ordered cilantro green curry halibut with jasmine rice. It was an amazing combination of textures and tastes, each mouthful a supernova of subtleties...the chef really knew what he was doing to be able to impart such an experience to another person through food. Every mouthful of fish, cooked so as to melt in your mouth, along with some of the rice and a small aliquot of sauce invited a silent pause of, no exaggeration, dumbfounded ecstasy during which the head instinctively inclined itself at an unnatural angle to deepen the mindfulness of what was going on in the mouth. This was followed by an exclamation of delight and satisfaction, mostly contained so as to not overdo it with my wife, Myla, who had ordered something else. There was also a sensuous lingering after each mouthful with the swirling, explosive blending of refined tastes that was the source of such pleasure, mildly sweet, a touch of coconut milk aroma, and intensely peppered, but somehow not too much. Again, ultimately it is impossible for me to describe it. I guess that is why we eat delicious food, because just reading about it, even if the writer is gifted, may conjure up hunger, but it will never satisfy that hunger or give us the actual flavor itself. For that we have to take it into our mouths ourselves and taste it in order to know it. Here the tasting is the knowing.

When we taste with such care and attention, even the simplest of foods provide a universe of sensory experience. One bite of apple, banana, bread, cheese, one bite of anything is a whole universe of surprising tastes if we can be awake to them. Maybe that is why even the simplest of foods, even canned peas or sardines, taste better, it seems, when we are on the trail or camping, outside of our normal framework for experiencing the world.

And that is why eating a raisin is usually the first meditation practice we offer people in MBSR (mindfulness-based stress reduction). Eating dispels all previous concepts we may be harboring about meditation. It immediately places it in the realm of the ordinary, the everyday, the world you already know but are now going to know differently. Eating one raisin very very slowly invites you to drop right into the knowing in ways that are effortless, totally natural, and entirely beyond words and thinking. It is an invitation that is unusual only in that we tend to eat so automatically and unconsciously. Such an exercise, just eating, just chewing, just tasting, delivers wakefulness immediately: there is in this moment only tasting. Everything else is merely words and therefore thinking—once removed at least from present-moment experience, from tasting itself, and knowing intimately, savoring, the tastescape in the mouth.

Yet I imagine, coming back to the green curry halibut, that the chef might have something interesting and revealing to say about his creations. Tasting this dish mouthful after delicious mouthful, it was as if I were all of a sudden at a wine tasting and had been given some two-hundred-year-old Bordeaux costing hundreds of dollars. I might enjoy it, but how could I appreciate, never mind give voice to all its ineluctable virtues, or even understand them listening to someone else, without being a connoisseur of wines?

And what would that be? Just someone with experience, who has, literally, "become familiar" through paying attention to a particular field of experience (from the Latin, *cognoscere*, to know). So, in attending to the tastescape by bringing mindfulness to what we are actually putting in our mouths and tasting, we are becoming connoisseurs not only of what we are eating, but of who is doing the eating in the first place. It is all part of this particular field of awareness.

Let's actually give some thought to eating for a moment. After breathing, eating is just about as basic as it gets for living organisms. We cannot sustain ourselves without eating, and the drives to satisfy that daily need for sustenance, in particular hunger and thirst, along with the discrimination of taste, which in the wild reduced the chances of poisoning ourselves out of desperation when hungry or thirsty, require daily satisfaction.

In hunting-and-gathering societies, almost all the energy of every able-bodied person went into procuring food. In agricultural societies, where the majority of food is grown and raised rather than hunted and gathered, a huge amount of energy in the society still goes into food production. Nevertheless, agriculture and the raising of animals over time, at least in locations where the environment was conducive to it, provided surpluses of food that allowed for a growing complexity within social groups, the appearance of cities and civil society, wherein not everybody devoted their energies to food production or distribution, even though everybody in the society has to eat to stay alive. This trend has obviously continued and has become even more the case in industrial and postindustrial societies. Thus, our relationship to food over the past ten thousand years has changed dramatically, including the ease of procurement, preservation, storage, distribution, varieties of food available to us, its quality and nutritive value, and the ubiquity of it. From that have arisen many ways in which we who do not grow or catch our own food take both food and eating for granted, and we live very far from the basic need to find food when it is scarce or difficult to procure.

Nevertheless, eating is still just as basic to our survival, each and every one of us, as to prehistoric societies, so we live with a kind of tension of non-recognition and non-appreciation that can be quite bizarre. Thus eating has become increasingly separated from survival and maintenance of life in our consciousness. For the most part, we eat with great automaticity and little insight into its critical importance for us in sustaining life, and also in sustaining health. We are driven far more by desire than by need, our relationships to food shaped by social pressures, the advertising industry, agribusiness, food processing, and by conditioned taste preferences and portion sizes that, in first world countries and particularly the United States, have led to a virtual epidemic of obesity over little more than a decade.

*

I have eaten one raisin very very slowly with a lot of people over the years, and so have become somewhat identified in people's minds with raisins, enough to sometimes feel like protesting: "It's not about the raisin." The raisin is merely an occasion to explore the tastescape and our relationship to the whole domain of eating, which we usually engage in with considerable automaticity and often stunningly little awareness of what or how we are eating, how fast we are eating, what our food actually tastes like, and when our body is telling us it is time to stop. And beyond eating, of course, the raisin is also an occasion for us to investigate the nature of our own mind and body. For that matter, what we experience with the raisin can and often does reveal important elements of our relationship with the entire world.

Our eating is often driven by rather primordial urges and accompanied by equally primordial and extremely unconscious behaviors. I know from firsthand experience that becoming conscious of how we eat, and whether we are truly tasting anything at all, is one of the most difficult of all mindfulness practices, even though at first blush it seems self-evident and easy. But the habit patterns surrounding self-feeding run very deep, and as we just observed, there really is a primordial element to them. Just think: we feed ourselves, and we have all had to learn to do it. And we do it all the time, not just to sustain our lives, but often out of sheer habit, and the urge to satisfy cravings that have little to do with real nourishment and often stem more from emotional discomfort than any actual hunger. Of course, sharing food in the company of family and friends is one of the most basic, profound, and satisfying vehicles of social connectedness. It feeds other needs that also run very deep in us.

One way we know the world and are in touch with it is through the mouth and via the tongue, through its fine-tuned ability to distinguish textures as well as through tasting. As already noted, the tongue is relatively large in the somatosensory homunculus (see *The Healing Power of Mindfulness*, "Homunculus"), reflecting its importance as a vehicle for knowing the world, well beyond the specialized sense of taste. As babies, we all put things in our mouths. That was a primary and very direct way to explore what things were. Rocks are hard. Sand is gritty. Blueberries are squooshy. Everything has its own unique texture and feel in the mouth.

When we bring awareness intentionally into the mouth as we are chewing one raisin, after having looked at it for some time and have actually seen it beyond our concepts and opinions about it, the very taste itself tends to explode into our mouths and into our minds with a surprising novelty that can be quite revealing...a universe of sensations, all unfolding and mixing together in every moment. And it doesn't have to be a raisin. If we slow down a bit, we can intentionally bring awareness to tasting anything we are eating, to be with this mouthful of food and really taste it, chew it, and know it before we swallow it.

It is said that taste, perhaps closely coupled with smell, is the sense that is most unmistakably evocative of memories. One broadly known literary passage evoking this power of the sense of taste over memory comes from Marcel Proust's *Remembrance of Things Past*.

> The sight of the little madeleine had recalled nothing to my mind before I tasted it...[but] as soon as I had recognized the taste of the piece of madeleine soaked in her decoction of lime-blossom which my aunt used to give me...immediately the old grey house upon the street,

where her room was, rose up like a stage set to attach itself
to the little pavilion opening on to the garden which had
been built out behind it for my parents.

Let's keep this in mind, to be returned to later when we explore
the intimate links between the brain, our inward and outward
senses, our memories, and awareness itself.

MINDSCAPE

Landscape, lightscape, soundscape, touchscape, smellscape, tastescape, ultimately it all comes down to what we could call, by extension, *mindscape*. Without the discerning capacity of our minds, there would be no knowing of any landscape, inner or outer. When we become aware, when we rest in the knowing, we are resting in the deep essence of the mindscape, in the vast empty spaciousness that is awareness itself. It is its own sense. Perhaps the ultimate sense in that it can amplify the texture of all the others. And one that, as with our other senses, we can be aware of—in other words, we can cultivate awareness of awareness itself, and therefore access it in new and profoundly beneficial and transformative ways.

It is neither particularly easy nor particularly difficult to come by or inhabit the domain of awareness of our own mindscape. All we need is motivation, and perhaps to have it pointed out to us in the first place as worthy of intimacy. It is precisely the systematic cultivation of mindfulness that shows us ways to be available to the mindscape, to taste it, to smell it, to inhabit it, to be it, and thus make it maximally available to us.

Dropping in in any moment and dwelling here in awareness, fully awake to the entire field of experience however large or narrow we have set the lens, we readily observe that every aspect of experience comes and goes. No arising is permanent, no arising endures. Sights, sounds, sensations in the body, including of this in-breath and this out-breath, smells, tastes, perceptions, impulses, thoughts, emotions, moods, opinions, preferences, aversions, more opinions, all come and go, fluxing, changing constantly, offering us countless and rich opportunities to see into impermanence and our own habits of wanting and clinging.

In any moment, we can see, hear, touch, smell, taste, and know things as they are. It is not some ideal that we are striving for. Rather, it is the rich and multidimensional, multi-textured, kaleidoscopic reality of a momentary experience of being alive— complex yes, and yet so simple that it can be inhabited...if we bring awareness to it.

When we know something of the mindscape through a sustained cultivating of intimacy and familiarization with how things actually are in its domain, we are better able, in any and every moment, to let go of our fears that things will not work out for us (the future), and to let go of our various strivings to make sure that they will work out the way we want by subtly or not so subtly attempting to force them to (again the future).

In that moment, in any such moment, the spaciousness of awareness that we know and have tasted in our practice once it develops some stability and consistency, or that we have at least caught an occasional whiff of, can rotate our orientation in the mindscape to an acknowledgment if not a full acceptance of things as they are. In any moment, then, we might actually come in touch with our own wholeness, our own beauty, beyond name and form, beyond appearance, beyond liking and disliking, beyond good and bad. Here, and only here, is peace to be found. Here, and only here, can we contribute our wisdom, our energies, and our love to those we love and to the world. And we do that through *embodying* our intimacy with the mindscape. So we could say that the mindscape includes the *bodyscape,* the realm of all the senses, the body itself, and vice versa. Mysteriously, the mindscape is utterly embodied, and thus, intrinsically compassionate as well as wise. Why? Because of the boundless, all-inclusive nature of awareness itself, far beyond our body, driving an inevitable recognition of universal interconnectedness, and thus of self in other and other in self.

That element of intrinsic compassion within awareness doesn't mean, by the way, that in any particular moment, depending on various causes and conditions, there won't be conflict and a lack of acceptance, or a rending and pulling in your mind or in your life. There may very well be. That is as much a part of the mindscape of human beings, even those who practice mindfulness, as anything else. But, there may very well also be a gradual shift in the balance over time, from more inner conflict to more equanimity, from more anger to more compassion, from predominantly seeing only appearances to a deeper apprehending of the actuality of things. Or this may be so at times, and not so at other times. In any moment, there might be a degree of equanimity, a degree of compassion for yourself or for others, a degree of insight, and those need to be noted and honored along with all the other creatures inhabiting this inner landscape. In the end, there is no ideal here that needs reaching for. The mindscape is just and always as it is. The challenge is, can we know it? Can we not be caught by it? Can we be free of it? Can we be free in it? This is where the ongoing cultivation of intimacy with our moments comes in, inclining us in the direction of greater wakefulness and thus, the option of wise agency when we do act or take a stand.

NOWSCAPE

Everything that unfolds unfolds now, and so might be said to unfold in the *nowscape*. We've already observed how nature unfolds only and always in the now. The trees are growing now. The birds are flying through the air or sitting in the branches only now. The rivers and the mountains are in the now. The ocean is in the now. The planet itself is turning now. One physicist, writing about Einstein and time, observed that change in something is the way we measure time, and anything that changes in a regular way can therefore be called a clock. In fact, it is more accurate to be saying that change is the way we measure time than to say that time is the way we measure change, since time is in and of itself such a mystery. Everything changes, and so there is time. Everything changes, and so we experience time. Everything changes, and so we can experience change by stepping outside of time for a moment, and becoming intimate with what is, beyond the abstraction that is the mystery of time.

Time flows, time is passing, but we do not know what time is. And for us, when we ask what time it is, there is only one answer, and it shapes the moment no matter what Big Ben or your alarm clock or your watch, or the Grand Canyon, is telling you. Guess what? Once again, it is now.

The tiniest bit of reflection will make it evident to you that the present moment is the only moment we ever have in which to be alive. Perhaps that realization, seemingly so self-apparent and trivial, needs to sink in and drop deep down into our psyche, into the wellspring of our own hearts. But it is actually very hard to take it in fully, to really fathom it. There is no time other than now. We are not, contrary to what we think, "going" anywhere. Life will never be more rich in some other moment than it is in this one. Although we may imagine that some future moment will be more pleasant, or less, than this one, we can't really know. But whatever the future brings, it will not be what you expect, or what you think, and when it comes, it will be now too. It too will be a moment that can be very easily missed, just as easily missed as this one. And it too will be subject to continual change and the vagaries of all the causes and conditions that gave rise to it in previous moments.

In that sense, wherever we go, wherever we are, whatever is happening, and no matter what time it is or what the calendar says, we always have only moments to live.

And so, we might be drawn, somehow, to make the best use of our moments that we can, while we can, to be available to them. At first, that usually requires making an effort to pay attention in and to the present moment. Why? Because it is so quickly gone, and because it is so easy to get caught up in the landscapes of the senses and the mind and fixated on their various inhabitants and energies and very quickly lose touch with ourselves, with others, and with the world. We can spin off into the future, rail about the past, think that things will be OK someday provided this happens and that doesn't happen, all of which may be true to one degree or another, but it still has you missing your life, and in a sense, all life.

You could think of that as the Great Escape. We exit from the sensescapes and the mindscape, from the nowscape, in our desperate attempts to *escape*. It is a maneuver we engage in all too frequently, whenever things are not to our liking...and, ironically, even when they are. So we can either inhabit the inner and outer landscapes of the mind and the body and the world, not really separate, or we can pursue the Great Escape and forget that our lives are as continually and wonderfully pregnant with possibility as they are, even in the most difficult and trying of times. And, that they are not to be missed.

The senses can wake us up, and they can also lull us to sleep. The mind can wake us up, or it too can lull us to sleep. The senses unfold only in the present, but in an instant they can catapult us into memory or into anticipation, and thus into endless and usually unhelpful preoccupation with the past, what did or didn't happen and how that all affects "me" now; or obsession with the future and all its worrying and planning for a better now later, when we might let down and be who we really are but don't have time to be now.

In the process, the present moment, the only moment we have, can get severely squeezed, to the point of hardly ever being seen or felt or known, or for that matter, used. It is only mindfulness that can reconstitute it and return us to it and it to us, for indeed, there is no difference between these. We and the nowscape are always here and never two. But this actuality can only be felt. It cannot be fathomed by thought alone because lived, experiential dimensions of it get denatured in the very process of thinking. It cannot be reduced to thought because it cannot be reduced at all. Now is that fundamental. And so are you.

This is not to say that we cannot or should not care about the future and work hard for necessary social change, for greater justice and economic freedom, for greater ecological balance and for a more peaceful world for all sentient beings. Nor does it mean that we should become apathetic and not work to accomplish our purposes and realize our visions and our dreams. It does not mean that we cannot continue to work at learning, growing, healing, and mobilizing our creative imagination and energies for our own benefit and happiness, as well as for the contributions we make to the worlds of others by the work we do and just by loving life. It is rather that if we, understandably, desire the future to be different, either on the large national, international, social, or geopolitical scale of things or in terms of improving our own life situation and that of our community, or just getting done what most needs getting done, there is only one time we ever have to influence that future.

For now is already the future and it is already here. Now is the future of the previous moment just past, and the future of all those moments that were before that one. Remember back in your own life for a moment, to when you were a child, or an adolescent, or a young adult, or to any other period already gone. This is that future. The you you were hoping to become, it is you. Right here. Right now. You are it. Don't like it? Who doesn't like it? Who is even thinking that? And who wants "you" to be better, to have turned out some other way? Is that you you too? Wake up! This is it. You have already turned out.

But, and it is a big but, do you know who you are fully, right now, in this moment? That is the question. That is what mindfulness is all about, because this really is it. Mindfulness is an ongoing inhabiting of the nowscape. It is a wakefulness that lies beyond being continually caught in liking and disliking, wanting and rejecting, and in destructive and unexamined emotional habits and thought patterns, no matter how important the issue, no matter how little or how great the stakes. Imagine working in and for the world from such a vantage point, with that kind of perspective.

That might be a worthy assignment, a worthy challenge we could proffer ourselves and practice embodying in the world in this very moment, right here, today.

Each moment of now is what we could call a branch point. We do not know what will happen next. The present moment is pregnant with possibility and potential. When we are mindful now, no matter what we are doing or saying or working on or experiencing, the next moment is influenced by our presence of mind, and is thus different from how it would have been had we not been paying attention, had we been caught up in some whirlpool or other within the mind or body or the outer landscape. So, if we wish to take care of the future that, when we get there, will also be now, the only way we can do that is to take care of this future of all past moments and efforts, namely, the present. The only way we can do that is to recognize each moment as a branch point and realize that it makes all the difference in how the world, your world, and your one wild and precious life, will unfold. We take care of the future best by taking care of the present now.

This should be ample incentive to act with integrity and presence and with kindness and compassion for ourselves and for others. Arriving someplace more desirable at some future time is an illusion. This is it.

Not a bad reason to *practice* being here for it. That is what formal meditation practice, which we will now visit in Part 2, is all about.

Embracing Formal Practice

Tasting Mindfulness

Have you ever had the experience of stopping so completely,
of being in your body so completely,
of being in your life so completely,
that what you knew and what you didn't know,
that what had been and what was yet to come,
and the way things are right now
no longer held even the slightest hint of anxiety or discord?
It would be a moment of complete presence, beyond striving, beyond mere
    acceptance,
beyond the desire to escape or fix anything or plunge ahead,
a moment of pure being, no longer in time,
a moment of pure seeing, pure feeling,
a moment in which life simply is,
and that "isness" grabs you by all your senses,
all your memories, by your very genes,
by your loves, and
welcomes you home.

Lying Down Meditations

The most important thing to keep in mind when practicing meditation lying down is that, as with every aspect of the cultivation and embodiment of mindfulness, it is about falling awake.

But because whenever we lie down there is always the "occupational hazard" of falling asleep, we actually have to work at remembering to *fall awake* in the face of a not-insignificant possibility that we might drift into drowsiness and unawareness and fall asleep. With ongoing practice, however, it is actually possible to train yourself and thereby learn to fall awake, both in the conventional sense of not falling asleep or getting sleepy, and also in the deeper sense of being utterly present in awareness.

There are many virtues to meditating lying down. For one, in the early stages of meditation practice, it may be more comfortable if you are lying down rather than sitting, and you can probably be still for longer periods of time. Then, because we lie down when we sleep, it gives us several built-in occasions every day for touching base with ourselves, one before we fall asleep at the end of the day, and one in the morning as we are waking up. These are perfect occasions to introduce a stretch of formal meditation practice into your day, whether for just a few minutes or for longer, *especially* when waking up in the morning. Also, when the body is stretched out, particularly lying on your back, it is in general fairly easy to feel your belly moving with the breath, rising and expanding on the in-breaths and falling and deflating on the out-breaths. This position also gives us a sense of being held up, buoyed, supported by whatever surface we are lying on. We can surrender completely to the embrace of gravity, and let go into the floor or mat or bed and let it do the work of holding us up. Sometimes in this position, it can feel like you are floating, and that experience can be very pleasant and increase your motivation for taking up residency in your body and in the present moment.

What's more, the surrender of the body to gravity can entrain the mind into the spirit of what we might call unconditional surrender, not to some external threat to our well-being, but to a full inhabiting of the present moment, independent of any conditions we may find ourselves in. In practicing dropping into the embrace of gravity itself, we are more motivated and more willing to drop unconditionally into now, to bring a radical and openhearted acceptance to whatever we find is going on in our minds or bodies and in our lives in any moment or on any given day, in a word, to let be and let go.

When formally cultivating mindfulness while lying down, whether we are in bed or on the floor, it can be especially valuable to intentionally adopt what is known in yoga as the corpse pose, lying on our backs with our arms alongside the body and the feet falling away from each other. There is nothing particularly maudlin about thinking of it as the corpse pose. It is simply a reminder that we can intentionally die to the past and die to the future, and thus give ourselves over to the present moment and to the life expressing itself in us now. Because you are indeed kind of corpse-like in the way you are lying, it is easy in this posture to intentionally evoke an attitude of dying inwardly to the ordinary preoccupations of the mind and the world for a time at least, and opening to the richness of this moment. But that said, of course you can practice mindfulness in any lying down posture that you care to, such as curled up lying on your side, or lying on your belly. Every posture has its own unique energies and challenges, and every posture is a perfect posture for meeting the present moment with embodied wakefulness and openheartedness. And of course, whatever posture you choose to adopt, there are many different ways to practice, and many different practices to bring to bear on the present moment.

*

So, lying on a comfortable padded surface, either on a rug or pad on the floor, or in bed or on a couch, we might at first give ourselves over to the experience of being here like this, in this posture, whatever it is. In part, this might entail opening to the soundscape and letting it speak, hearing whatever is here to be heard, as if we had died and were now merely overhearing the world going on, only now without us. With this attitude and orientation, we may hear sounds and sense the spaces between them in an entirely new way. Alternatively, you may notice at first that you haven't been hearing any sounds at all, so absorbed have you been in the roar of sensations fluxing in the body or in what you might call mental noise, the thoughts racing incessantly through your head.

The entire meditation could be dedicated simply to being with hearing, bringing our attention back to hearing over and over again when it wanders off, and perhaps inquiring in a nondiscursive way as to "Who is hearing?" This is an extremely powerful way to practice...the coming to our senses through the sense of hearing.

Or, we might allow hearing to be one aspect of our lived experience, which of course it is, and practice with an open, more undirected spaciousness of attention that drinks in sensations and perceptions emanating from all the senses at once, inwardly and outwardly, as they arise moment by moment. And since we are looking at the mind as a sixth sense organ of sorts, the field of awareness would naturally include any and all mental phenomena as well. This practice of undirected spaciousness of attention, which we shall explore in more detail later, is called *choiceless awareness*.

Alternatively we might practice just attending solely to the sensations of breathing, or being with sensations in specific regions of the body, or with an all-embracing sense of the body as a whole. As part of this last practice, we might either include or choose to feature the skin, feeling the entirety of the envelope of the body, tuning to whatever sensations are present as we lie here, and aware of how they are changing. We might also tune to a sense of the air around the body, bathing the body, enveloping the body, breathing the body, and perhaps even imagining the skin itself breathing.

We can also just dwell in the watching of our thoughts and the emotional "charges" that they carry, whether positive, negative, or neutral, whether relatively strong or relatively weak, featuring them center stage in the field of awareness while we let all the other aspects of the present moment recede into the wings. Alternatively, we can place one object of attention in the foreground for a period of time, then allow it to recede into the background as we bring forth some other aspect of the field of awareness and feature it center stage in the field of awareness.

As you can see, the mindfulness palette is a big one, whatever our posture. It is continually inviting us to make use of various methods and scaffolding and honor how necessary and important they are in the cultivation and deepening of awareness, equanimity, and non-attachment. At the same time, as we have seen, we can keep in mind and continually "re-mind" ourselves that we can rest in awareness with any object of attention, the breath, various aspects of the body, with sensations and perceptions, with the myriad thoughts and feelings that flux through our minds, or in a vast, boundless, choiceless, open awareness beyond all doing, and just be the knowing that is awareness itself.

In making such choices, we can also choose to keep our eyes open or closed. If we keep them open in the corpse posture, we simply drink in through the eyes whatever is above us, usually a ceiling of some kind. Of course, if you are lying in a meadow on a warm clear day, gazing up at clouds for hours at a time is a meditation in its own right, as is gazing up into a tree you might be lying beneath. And of course, keeping the eyes open can be especially helpful and effective in moments of drowsiness and fatigue.

But it is also quite wonderful to practice lying down meditation with the eyes closed. Many people find it helpful in refining the awareness of the internal landscape of the body and the mind to keep the eyes closed. They find that it enhances the inward focus and concentration. That is something that you can decide for yourself, and something to experiment with from time to time intentionally.

There is no one right way to practice. Some traditions practice with eyes open, others with eyes closed. Sometimes our choice will be dictated by the circumstances of the moment and how we are feeling. But it is best in the early years of meditation to practice primarily one way or the other so that we can come to know the depths of the choice we have made, and not simply flit back and forth from one to the other depending on our mood.

As we have noted, it is very valuable to practice lying down meditation before falling asleep and again right away upon waking up. Sandwiching the day in this way, you get to prime and refine your commitment to mindfulness first thing in the morning before even getting out of bed. This can have a profoundly positive and beneficial effect on the entirety of your day, turning the whole of it into one opportunity to practice after another, literally moment by moment. You might even formulate the intention, before getting out of bed, that the entire day will be one seamless meditation on being present in, with, and to your life, as it is and as it is unfolding, bringing to each moment an openhearted curiosity and clarity. That awareness might then extend itself to the very process of the body getting itself out of bed, of brushing your teeth, of taking a shower,* and on through whatever you are engaging in that day. Then, lying in bed at the end of the day, you might experience the body and the mind and how they are in the aftermath of all that has transpired, resting in a felt sense of the body as a whole, and an open spaciousness of mind, beyond judging what was "good" and what was "bad" about the day. Lying here, we can tune in to a sense

---

* As an easily accessible example of how readily the mind drifts off into stories and mental noise and loses touch with the body and with the actuality of the present moment, I often suggest to people that the next time they are taking a shower, they might check and see if they are in the shower. It is not uncommon to find that you are not in the shower at all, but in a meeting with your colleagues that hasn't happened yet, for instance. Actually, in that moment, the whole meeting could be said to be in the shower with you. Meanwhile you may be missing the experience of the water on your skin and pretty much everything else about that moment.

of the body as a whole, and into our wholeness of being and feel how we are nested in larger and larger spheres of wholeness and relationality extending outward far beyond ourselves. In this way, we can gradually let go of all that has come before and welcome sleep as it comes over us.

In addition to practicing right before going to sleep and right after waking up (after all, why not finish the job and wake up completely before getting out of bed each morning?), lying down meditation can be practiced at any time, using any of the approaches outlined above. Ultimately, as with all meditation, it is about dropping in on this moment as it is and resting in awareness, outside of time, discerning from moment to moment how things actually are.

There are times when I feel a great urge to get on the floor or on the bed and meditate lying down rather than sitting or in some other posture. Just getting down on the floor for a while, or on the earth for that matter, can change your whole orientation toward the moment and the day and what is transpiring. It can slow down or stop the forward momentum of the head and all its drivenness and help you to recalibrate and be more embodied in whatever you are dealing with. It can also enlarge your view of your own mind and body in that moment and how they are responding to what is going on. And, of course, lying down meditation can be profoundly valuable when you are sick in bed for any reason, or in the hospital, or undergoing difficult diagnostic procedures that can take a long time, such as CAT scans and MRIs, which require you to lie down and be very still.

We can turn almost any situation in which we are lying down into an opportunity to practice, and in doing so, discover hidden dimensions of our own life and new possibilities for learning and growing and healing and for transformation, nested right inside the present moment, possibilities and insights that are much more likely to emerge when we are willing to show up and be with whatever is arising.

And then there is the body scan.

The body scan has proven to be an extremely powerful and healing form of meditation. It forms the core of the lying down practices that people train in in MBSR. It involves systematically sweeping through the body with the mind, bringing an affectionate, openhearted, interested attention to its various regions, customarily starting from the toes of the left foot and then moving through the entirety of the foot—the sole, the heel, the top of the foot—then up the left leg, including in turn the ankle, the shin and the calf, the knee and the kneecap, the thigh in its entirety, on the surface and deep, the groin and the left hip, then over to the toes of the right foot, the other regions of the foot, then up the right leg in the same manner as the left. From there, the focus moves into, successively, and slowly, the entirety of the pelvic region, including the hips again, the buttocks and the genitals, the lower back, the abdomen, and then the upper torso—the upper back, the chest and the ribs, the breasts, the heart and lungs and great vessels housed within the rib cage, the shoulder blades floating on the rib cage in back, all the way up to the collarbones and shoulders. From the shoulders, we move to the arms, usually doing them together, starting from the tips of the fingers and thumbs and moving successively through the fingers, the palms and backs of the hands, the wrists, forearms, elbows, upper arms, armpits, and shoulders again. Then we move into the neck and throat, and, finally, the face and head.

Along the way, we might tune in to some of the remarkable

anatomical structures, biological functions, and more poetic, metaphorical, and emotional dimensions of the various regions of the
body and each region's particular individual history and potential:
whether it is the ability of the feet to hold us up; the sexual and
generative energies of the genitals; in women, the capacity to give
birth and the memories of pregnancies and births for those who
have had the experience; the eliminative and purifying functions
associated with the bladder, kidneys, and bowels; the digestive fires
of the abdomen and its role in breathing and in grounding us in the
physical center of gravity of the body; the stresses and triumphs of
the lower back in carrying us upright in the gravitational field; the
radiant potential inherent in the solar plexus; the chest as the location of the metaphorical as well as the physical heart (we speak, for
instance, of being lighthearted, heavyhearted, hard-hearted, bro-
kenhearted, warm-hearted, glad-hearted, and of "getting things
off our chests"); the huge mobility of the shoulders; the beauty
of the hands and arms; the remarkable structures and functions
of the larynx, which allow us, in combination with the lungs and
the tongue, the lips and the mouth, to express what is in our hearts
and on our minds in speech and in song; how hard the face works
to convey what we are feeling or hide what we are feeling, and
the quiet dignity of the human face in repose; and the remarkable, ever-changing architecture and capacities of the human brain
(the most complex arrangement of matter in the known-by-us
universe, housed right under the vault of the cranium) and nervous system. Any or all of these might be embedded within our
appreciation of the body as we sweep through it with affectionate
attention and mindful awareness, not shunning thoughts about the
body or feelings about it either, but simply holding it all in awareness, "underneath thinking."

The body scan can be undertaken and practiced with great precision and detail, visualizing the various regions in your mind's eye one by one as you "inhabit" them with awareness and linger with them, outside of time. That might include sensing how the breath is moving in and through each region (which of course it does, because the breath energy reaches and bathes each and every region through the vehicle of the oxygenated blood). If you are doing it on your own, without guidance from a CD, download, or app, and you have the time and the inclination, you can proceed at your own leisurely pace, taking time to inhabit each region and cultivate a deep intimacy with it as it is in that moment through your breath and through the direct, moment-to-moment attending to the raw sensations emanating from it. When ready, you can then let it be and let go of it as you choose to move on to the next region.

Our patients in the MBSR Clinic practice the body scan forty-five minutes a day, at least six days per week for the first two weeks of the program, using audio guidance voiced by their instructor. In the weeks that follow, they keep practicing the body scan, but now alternating it first with mindful yoga and then later, with formal sitting meditation, also guided by their instructor. Having the body scan at the core of your mindfulness practice in the early stages is recommended, especially if you are faced with chronic health conditions and/or chronic pain of any kind. That said, the body scan is not for everybody, nor is it is always the meditation of choice even for those who love it. But it is extremely useful and good to know about and practice from time to time, whatever your circumstances or condition. If you think of your body as a musical instrument, the body scan is a way of tuning it. If you think of it as a universe, the body scan is a way to come to know it. If you think of your body as a house, the body scan is a way to throw open all the windows and doors and let the fresh air of awareness sweep it clean.

You can also scan your body much more quickly, depending on your time constraints and the situation you find yourself in. You can do a one in-breath one out-breath body scan, or a one-, two-, five-, ten-, or twenty-minute body scan. The level of precision and detail will of course vary depending on how quickly you move through the body, but each speed has its virtues, and ultimately, it is about being in touch with the whole of your being and your body in any and every way you can, outside of time altogether.

You can practice body scans, long or short, lying in bed at night or in the morning. You can also practice them sitting or even standing. There are countless creative ways to bring the body scan or any other lying down meditation into your life. If you make use of any of them, it is highly likely that you will find that they will bring new life to you, and bring you to a new appreciation for your body and how much it can serve as a vehicle for embodying here and now what is deepest and best in yourself, including your dignity, your beauty, your vitality, and your mind when it is open and undisturbed.

Once again, I cannot recommend lying down meditations highly enough, especially in bed in the morning. Conventionally speaking, when we get out of bed in the morning, we call it waking up. But are we really? We may still be half-asleep and already running on autopilot. Why not check in in that very moment and see if we don't need to actually finish the job? Why not make sure that you are fully awake and aware and in touch with the body and not so much lost in thought and already driven by what your calendar has in store for you before your feet hit the floor and you move into your day? That is an extremely powerful practice, and can easily become a way of being that extends your awareness powerfully throughout the day and into the night. It might even be worth making some extra time for it, setting the alarm clock a bit earlier perhaps, and building a time for falling completely awake into your morning routine.

SITTING MEDITATIONS

Like lying down meditations, there are many different ways to cultivate mindfulness while sitting. Ultimately, they all boil down to skillful ways for dwelling with what is in the landscape of the present moment, and being with and knowing things as they actually are. Sounds simple. And it is. At the same time, there is nothing casual about sitting meditation, just as there is nothing casual about any other form of practice. We can and need to be kind and gentle with ourselves, and at the same time sit as if our lives depended on it. Because, when it comes right down to it, they surely do.

But in order to understand this, we have to understand what it means to sit. It doesn't just mean to be seated. It means taking your seat in and in relationship with the present moment. It means taking a stand in your life, sitting. That is why adopting and maintaining a posture that embodies dignity—whatever that means to you—is so helpful in the formal practice of sitting. The embodiment of dignity inwardly and outwardly immediately reflects and radiates the sovereignty of your life, that you are who and what you are—beyond all words, concepts, and descriptions, and beyond what anybody else thinks about you, or even what *you* think about you. It is a dignity without self-assertion—not driving forward *toward* anything, nor recoiling *from* anything—a balancing in sheer presence, a presencing.

Even if you don't always feel it, it is helpful to come to sitting practice as if it were a radical act of love just to sit in this way—love for yourself, love for others, love for the world, love for silence and for insight, love for compassion, love for what is most important. Over time, you will come to see that it is so in ways that go far deeper than these words or any concepts you may have about practice.

From this perspective, what we mean by "sitting" can be practiced in any posture, including lying down or standing. Because it is the inner orientation that is being spoken of, not literally whether you are seated or not. It is the mind that is "sitting."

But that being said, on a purely literal level, formal sitting practice has much to recommend it, not the least of which is its great potential stability, the reduced likelihood, compared to lying down, that you will fall asleep, and the reduced likelihood, compared to standing, that you will be challenged by fatigue from maintaining the posture itself. For sitting, especially when you learn to establish yourself in a stable posture as economically as possible from the point of view of muscular effort, supports your capacity to practice mindfulness with great concentration and with stable, penetrative, unwavering qualities of mind and body.

In terms of body posture, the greatest stability comes from sitting on the floor in one of a number of cross-legged positions, supported by a meditation cushion or bench that raises your buttocks off the floor to an appropriate degree.* Since sitting on the floor is

---

* Useful tip if sitting on a meditation cushion (zafu): sit on the forward third of it rather than dead-center on top of it. This allows your pelvis to tilt forward and encourages a slight but important forward-facing (lordotic) curve in the lower back.

not always congenial for people, especially at the beginning, and since ultimately the practice is not about the stability of the body but about the stability and openness and clarity of the mind and the sincerity of your motivation to practice, what you are sitting on is relatively unimportant. Even your physical posture is relatively unimportant. Sitting on a chair is an equally valid and powerful way to practice sitting meditation, especially if the chair has a straight back and supports your sitting in an erect upright position that embodies wakefulness and dignity. But let's keep in mind not to get too attached even to the concept of dignity, and of sitting a certain way. It is really the inner attitude that is most important here—not the outward posture.

Once established in a sitting posture, we simply give ourselves over to awareness of the present moment. The options are the same as for lying down meditations, and as with them, we can work with the eyes closed or open in any of these sitting practices as well.

Perhaps hearing is the most basic door into sitting meditation, since we have nothing to do other than to be aware of the sounds already arriving at our ears. Since everything is already happening, since we are already hearing, there is actually nothing to do other than to know it. The challenge is, *can* we know it? *Can* we sit here from moment to moment simply hearing what is here to be heard, without the elaborations and diversions of the ruminative, discursive mind? The answer is, for most of us, most of the time, "No, we can't." But we can investigate this very challenge. We can experiment with cultivating awareness of how out of touch we can be with such an obvious aspect of the present moment. So in this particular form of practice, we open our attention to the soundscape and sustain it within the soundscape as best we can, moment by moment by moment as we sit here. In the words of the Buddha, in the hearing there is only the heard. When the mind wanders, as it inevitably will, we note what is on our mind in that moment (which is always *this* moment when it occurs) or downstream from it in the moment when we finally realize we are no longer attending to sound. We note whatever is on our mind in *that* moment, and we do so as best we can without judgment or criticism, or without judging the judging and the criticizing if they do occur. Then and there, which is already now and here, we simply allow our awareness to include hearing once again, and thus allow hearing to resume its place as the primary locus of attention. We bring the mind back to hearing, over and over again, when it is carried off, distracted, or diverted away from hearing.

Another option, equally simple and accessible for people at the beginning stages of meditation practice, is to feature the breath as the primary object of attention rather than the soundscape, since the breath, like sound, is always present, and since, literally and metaphorically, you can't leave home without it. As with hearing, the invitation to attend to the experience of our own breathing from moment to moment may be simple as a concept but it is far from easy as a practice, especially in the sustaining of our attention on the breath. And as with hearing meditation, breath awareness is potentially as profound as any other form of meditation, since ultimately the mindfulness that is cultivated is the same and the insights that it has the potential to give rise to are also the same.

It is never the object of attention that is primary. It is always the *attending* itself. This is a key principle to keep in mind, whatever your practice, whatever object or objects of attention you have singled out. What we pay attention to, while important, is secondary. The various sense doors are all different entry points into awareness itself. The point is not to prefer one door to another, or to stand in the doorway and comment on it. Rather it is to enter the space of awareness and take up residency here, whatever doorway you choose to enter through.

The basic instructions for mindfulness of breathing are that, while maintaining the dignified sitting posture we have adopted as best we can, we focus on the breath sensations at a place in the body where they are most vivid, usually at the nostrils or at the abdomen. Then, to whatever degree we can manage it, we sustain our awareness of the feeling of the breath at the nostrils as it passes in and out of the body; or, alternatively, we sustain attending to the sensations associated with the rising and the falling of the belly with the in-breaths and the out-breaths.

When we find that the mind has wandered away from the primary object of our attention, as is bound to happen over and over again, we simply note what is on our mind at the moment we remember the breath and realize that we have not been in touch with it for some time. And we do so without judgment or self-condemnation, again, as best we can. We note that the realization that we are no longer with the breath is itself awareness, and so we are already back in the present moment. Importantly, we do not have to dispel or push away or even remember whatever it was that was preoccupying the mind the moment before. We simply allow the breath to once again resume its place as the primary object of our attention, since it has never not been here and is as available to us in this very moment as in any other.

Another powerful sitting meditation practice involves expanding the field of awareness to include sensations within the body, once you feel stable in either the breath awareness or in awareness of hearing, whichever you are using. This can include awareness of sensations in various parts of the body as they arise, perhaps dominate for a while, and then change over the course of a moment or over the course of an entire sitting, sensations such as discomfort in a knee, or in the lower back, a headache if it arises, or for that matter, subtle or vivid feelings of ease, comfort, and pleasure within the body. Sensations might include feelings of pressure and temperature at the points of contact of the body with the floor, or tingling, itching, pulsations, aching, throbbing, light touch from the air currents, warmth or coolness anywhere in the body, the possibilities are endless. They may also include significant degrees of physical discomfort or pain that might arise either from sitting without moving for extended periods of time, or from a particular medical condition. None of these has to be an impediment to developing or deepening your sitting meditation practice, although it is always important to err on the side of being conservative and not pushing beyond your limits of the moment. But, to whatever degree it is possible, we simply sit with an awareness of sensations within the body, whatever they are, noting them as pleasant, unpleasant, or neutral, noting their level of intensity, and as best we can not reacting emotionally to them or inflaming them with our preference for it to be another way so that our meditation might be "better" than what we are experiencing right now. In a word, we simply put out the red carpet for whatever sensations are arising in this moment and embrace them as they are, wherever they are, beneath the colorations of our likes and dislikes and our expectations for how things should be but aren't, all in the service of cultivating greater intimacy with the nowscape, which, as we've seen over and over again in so many ways, includes and is grounded in the body. In this way, we are cultivating an exquisite intimacy with the bodyscape and the sensations through which it makes itself known.

We can also practice sitting with a sense of the body as a whole sitting and breathing. This is a practice I find particularly congenial. Some traditions refer to it as whole body sitting. Here we open

to the subtle sensoria of proprioceptive and interoceptive knowing as well as to the more individual isolated sensations within the
body. Awareness now embraces the entirety of the body, including the skin, and the sitting posture itself. Within this sensory
field, any and all sensations, including all those mentioned previously, can be noted fluxing continuously throughout the body and
in the same way as before, simply opened to, known at the point
and moment of contact as pleasant, unpleasant, or neutral, and, to
whatever degree you can manage it, accepted as they are, however
they are, wherever they are.

In this practice, the breath and the body as a whole come
together (not that they are ever separate), are seen and felt and
known as one, and we simply rest here from moment to moment,
and of course, reestablish that condition over and over again when it
is lost to the distractions of the mind or to the incessant call of the
outer landscape.

As you can see, the process of expanding the field of awareness around the breath and the body as a whole sitting is virtually
limitless. We can include hearing, seeing (if our eyes are open), and
smelling as we sit here, either featuring them singly, or attending to
them all together as they unfold moment by moment. Yet the over-
all stance remains the same: resting in awareness itself and seeing, hearing, feeling, sensing, knowing whatever it is that is being
seen, heard, felt, sensed, or known in the moment of its arising, the
moment of its lingering, and the moment of its passing away. We
are the knowing because we align with that in us that is most fundamental, our capacity for awareness, for knowing itself, beyond
the conventional boundaries of name and form and concepts of
any kind.

In sitting meditation, we can also choose to allow the world
of somatic sensations, including the breath sensations, to recede

into the background, along with the soundscape and our other sensing modalities, as we feature center stage in the field of awareness some other particular aspect of our experience in the present moment, such as the thinking process itself and/or our emotions. Here we are attending to the activity of the mind itself as a sensory organ, in the same way that we can attend to the activity of the five more traditional senses and, in so doing, refine our familiarity and intimacy with it and how it functions to either enhance or suppress awareness.

In this practice, as we sit here, we simply bring our attention to thoughts as events in the field of awareness, arising and passing away in what can often feel like a gushing stream, torrent, or waterfall. As best we can, we note their content, the emotional charge they carry (again, pleasant, unpleasant, or neutral), and their evanescent and passing nature, while attempting, again, as best we can, not to be drawn into the content of any thought, which we will easily find will merely lead to another thought, image, memory, or fantasy, carrying us away in the stream of one thought proliferating into the next, rather than staying with the knowing frame in which all thoughts are seen with a degree of equanimity, discerned as events with content and emotional charge, and left alone to simply be what they are, momentary events arising, lingering, and dissolving in the mindscape, in the field of awareness itself.

Here, as implied by these verbal descriptions of the process, certain images may be helpful in supporting your practice as long as you don't cling to them or take them too literally. For instance, if we imagine our thoughts and emotions as a ceaseless river that is flowing endlessly, whether we are meditating or not, whether we are observing it or not, it can be helpful at times to think of the practice as an invitation to sit by the bank and listen to its endless bubbles, gurgles, and eddies, its voices, images, and stories, rather than be caught up in them and carried downstream. We can sit on the bank of our own mindstream, and by listening to its voices, come to know it, how it behaves, and what it carries in ways we never could if we are perpetually caught up in it. This is a direct and effective way to investigate the nature of the mind using your own mind as both the tool and the object of the investigation.

Another related image that people find useful is that of the cascading mind, as if the stream of our thoughts and emotions were flowing over a high cliff, producing a great waterfall. We can imagine that there is a cave behind the curtain of water and spray, within which we can sit and watch and listen to the stream of thoughts and emotions, perhaps perceiving at least some of them as individual water droplets, as discrete events within the chaotic complexity of falling water, individual events that can be seen and felt and known without falling into the gushing torrent itself and being carried away by it, without even getting soaked by the spray. We remain cozy and dry, just being with, just knowing each mind event, each bubble, as it appears, lingers, and dissolves.

Another image that may be helpful in attending mindfully to thoughts and emotions is that of observing an endless procession of cars on a street below, as if seen from behind a high window. Our assignment is to simply note dispassionately the car that is below the window in this moment. Since the cars may be old or new, fancy or plain, rare or common, electric or not, the mind may wind up thinking about one car long after it has passed, fantasizing about it, or wondering about it in relationship to other cars seen or unseen, or other car manufacturers, currently in business or long gone. If one car has sentimental value, for whatever reason, the mind might find its way into memories of pleasant or unpleasant family outings one had as a child, or leap to dreaming about the next car one hopes to buy, or reflecting on global warming and perhaps doing without an automobile. In any event, hundreds of cars may have gone by unnoticed because we were carried away by our preoccupation with one that happened to get the thought-stream going. Whenever that happens, we note as best we can what the chain of events was that carried us away. We note where we are now, and we pick up once again with the car that is front and center in our frame of reference right now. This is guaranteed to happen over and over again.

Whatever image or process you choose to employ, watching our thoughts and feelings is extremely difficult because they proliferate so wildly, and because, even though insubstantial and evanescent, they do fabricate our very reality, our story of who and what we are, and of what we care about and what has meaning for us; and because they come laden with emotional tie-ins that are none other than our mostly unexamined habits for insuring our survival and making sense of the world and our place in it.

As a consequence, we are usually very attached to many if not most of our thoughts and feelings, whatever they are, and simply relate to their content unquestioningly, as if it were the truth, hardly ever recognizing that thoughts and feelings are actually discrete events within the field of awareness, tiny and fleeting occurrences that are usually at least somewhat if not highly inaccurate and unreliable. Our thoughts may have a degree of relevance and accuracy at times, but often they are at least somewhat distorted by our self-centered and self-cherishing inclinations, such as our ambitions, our aversions, and our overriding tendency to ignore or be deluded by both our ambition and our aversions, and also perhaps by unacknowledged self-righteousness at times.

And then there is the practice of choiceless awareness.

Given that the field of awareness we have been cultivating

through the various practices described above is fundamentally limitless by nature, we can expand our awareness still further, beyond even attending specifically to the stream of our own thoughts and emotions arising and passing away in each moment. We can, instead, allow the field of awareness to be essentially infinite, boundless, like space itself, or like the sky, noting that it can include any and all aspects of our experience, interior and exterior, sensory, perceptual, somatic, emotional, cognitive as primary objects of attention, and that we can rest in this vast, sky-like field of awareness without choosing among or specifically featuring any of these particular occurrences. Instead, we allow them all to come and go, appear and disappear, as they will, and be known in their fullness from moment to moment within the nowscape.

This is the practice of what Krishnamurti called *choiceless awareness*, akin to the practice of *shikan-taza*, or "just sitting—nothing more" in Zen, and to *Dzogchen* in the Tibetan tradition. The Buddha called it the themeless concentration of awareness. The mind itself, once cultivated in this way, has the ability instantly to know and recognize what is arising, whatever it is, as it is arising, and instantly discern its true nature. With the arising, it is known non-conceptually by the mind itself, as if the sky knew the birds and the clouds and the moonlight within it. And in that knowing, with no attachment, no aversion, in that knowing in this very moment of now, the event, the sensation, the memory, the thought bubble in the stream, the feeling of hurt or sadness, or anger, or joy "self-liberates," as the Tibetans like to say, like touching a soap bubble, but with the mind, or, put differently, dissipates naturally in the knowing, like "writing on water."

*

This being human is a guest-house
Every morning a new arrival.

A joy, a depression, a meanness,
some momentary awareness comes
as an unexpected visitor.

Welcome and entertain them all!
Even if they're a crowd of sorrows,
who violently sweep your house
empty of its furniture,

still, treat each guest honorably.
He may be clearing you
out for some new delight.

The dark thought, the shame, the malice,
meet them at the door laughing,
and invite them in.

Be grateful for whoever comes,
because each has been sent
as a guide from beyond.

RUMI, "The Guest House"
Translated by Coleman Barks with John Moyne

STANDING MEDITATIONS

It is also possible to meditate standing up. Along with sitting, lying down, and walking, standing is one of the four classical postures for meditation.

In standing meditation, it is helpful to take our cues from trees because trees really know how to stand in one place for a very long time, at least relative to our brief lives. Yet they manage to be in the timeless present the whole time, however young or old they may be. So sometimes it can be helpful to just stand next to a favorite tree for a period of time and practice standing outside of time, hearing what the tree hears, experiencing the light the tree is experiencing, feeling the air the tree is feeling, standing on the soil the tree is standing on, inhabiting the moment the tree is inhabiting, and inhabiting, and inhabiting. . . .

As with all meditation practices, it helps to do this for longer than your first impulse to quit, to extend your standing out beyond the present limit of your patience, if just a little bit. It also helps, of course, if you are fully in your body, and perhaps imagining, if not feeling, that your feet are rooted to the ground and that your head is elevated with a sense of grace and ease toward the heavens (the Chinese character for man/person is a figure standing)—because between Heaven and Earth lies the domain in which the human unfolds.

This kind of standing is a conscious embodiment of standing in the midst of your own life, and thus, you could say, of taking a stand in your life. Your bearing, the carriage of your body, how evenly your weight is distributed on your feet, how you hold your head and how you hold your arms and your palms, even how long you are willing to remain, are all part of this huge gesture of mindfulness in the standing posture—so an awareness of these various elements can be quite useful. Of course, you stand however you can, but it is helpful to hold the intention to align yourself with the central, vertical axis of your very being, in other words, to stand with dignity. Such a bearing tends to clear and calm the mind and allows it to be more spacious and less contracted and congested.

And to this posture, you then bring or allow to unfurl a spacious awareness of the nowscape, including all the particular sensescapes and the mindscape of the present moment. Then, you give yourself over to simply being with what is unfolding, practicing as with sitting or lying down, with whatever subset of the scaffolding feels appropriate to you in this moment, including no scaffolding whatsoever, just this moment standing here, nothing more, being the knowing that awareness of standing here already is. This is choiceless awareness in the standing posture, a choiceless awareness that includes and subsumes the carriage of the body standing, breathing, hearing, seeing, touching, feeling, sensing, smelling, tasting, and knowing itself. You are not going anywhere. You are planted here, standing still, standing "firm in that which you are" in the words of the great Indian Sufi poet, Kabir.

Of course, standing meditation can be practiced anywhere, for any length of time, and not just in the vicinity of trees. You can practice waiting for elevators and while riding them, while waiting for buses and trains or for people you have arranged to meet at some appointed hour in some public place where it is not convenient to sit down. You can practice anytime, anywhere. You don't need to be waiting for anybody or anything. You can practice just standing for its own sake, not fidgeting, not moving much, a human being standing in his or her life. Just standing. Just being. Just being alive. Mountaintops, forests, beaches, jetties, porches, or a corner in any room in your house are all good places to practice standing and bearing witness to the unfolding of the world.

As usual, if it is to be mindful standing, a certain kind of rich intentionality and attention are required, whether they are invoked deliberately or emerge effortlessly in the moment. Certain poems speak of that attention, and its relationship to standing, and to trees, and the beauty of this present moment surrendered to fully.

*

Stand still. The trees ahead and the bushes beside you
Are not lost. Wherever you are is called Here,
And you must treat it as a powerful stranger,
Must ask permission to know it and be known.
The forest breathes. Listen. It answers,
I have made this place around you,
If you leave it you may come back again, saying Here.

No two trees are the same to Raven.
No two branches are the same to Wren.
If what a tree or a bush does is lost on you,

You are surely lost. Stand still. The forest knows
Where you are. You must let it find you.

DAVID WAGONER

*

My life is not this steeply sloping hour,
in which you see me hurrying.
Much stands behind me; I stand before it like a tree;
I am only one of my many mouths
and at that, the one that will be still the soonest.

I am the rest between two notes,
which are somehow always in discord
because death's note wants to climb over—
but in the dark interval, reconciled,
they stay here trembling.
                    And the song goes on, beautiful.

RAINER MARIA RILKE
Translated by Robert Bly

WALKING MEDITATIONS

Walking meditation is another door into the same room as sitting, lying down, or standing meditation. The spirit and orientation are the same, the scaffolding slightly different because we are moving. But ultimately, it is the same practice, only you are walking. But, and this is a big difference with regular walking, you are not going anywhere! Formal walking meditation is not about getting somewhere on foot. Instead, you are being with each step, fully here, where you actually are. You are not trying to get anywhere, even to the next step. There is no arriving, other than continually arriving in the present moment.

With walking, we have the opportunity to be in our bodies in a somewhat different way than when sitting or lying down. We can bring our attention to our feet and feel the contact of the foot with the floor or ground with every step, as if we were kissing the earth and the earth were kissing right back. We have already touched on the miracle of this, and the complete reciprocity of the touching. There are a myriad of sensations, proprioceptive and otherwise, one might include in the field of awareness.

Walking is a controlled falling forward, a process it took us a long time to master, and one that we often take completely for granted, forgetting just how wondrous and wonderful it is. So when the mind goes off, as it will do in walking meditation just as with any other practice, we take note of where it has gone, of what is presently on our mind, and then gently escort it back to this moment, this breath, and this step in the same ways we have already touched upon.

Since you are not going anywhere, it is best to minimize opportunities for self-distraction by walking slowly back and forth in a lane, over and over again. The lane doesn't have to be long. Ten paces one way, ten paces the other way would be fine. In any event, it is not a sightseeing tour of your environment. You keep your eyes soft and the gaze out in front of you. You do not have to look at your feet. They mysteriously know where they are, and awareness can inhabit them and be in touch with every part of the step cycle moment by moment by moment as well as with the whole of the body walking and breathing.

Walking meditation can be practiced at any number of different speeds, and that gives it lots of applications in daily living. In fact, we can easily go from mindful walking to mindful running, a wonderful practice in its own right. There, of course, we abandon the lane, as we can certainly do for long-distance and faster formal walks. But when we introduce formal mindful walking in MBSR, it is done extremely slowly, to damp down on our impulse to move quickly, as well as to refine our intimacy with the sensory dimensions of the experience of walking and how they are connected with the whole of the body walking and with the breath, to say nothing about having a better sense of what is going on in the mind.

We begin by standing and bringing awareness to the body as a whole standing at one end of the lane you have chosen for yourself. The field of awareness can include the entire nowscape. At a certain point, again, quite mysterious, we become aware of an impulse in the mind to initiate the process of walking by lifting one foot. So we become aware of the lifting, but not before we have let the *impulse* to lift the foot register, even as we saw in the raisin-eating meditation, when the instructions included being aware of the impulse to swallow before actually committing to the swallowing.

Beginning with lifting just the heel, we bring awareness to moving the entire foot and leg up and forward, and then to the placing of the foot on the ground, usually first with the heel. As the whole of this now forward foot comes down on the floor or ground, we note the shifting of the weight from the back foot through to the forward foot, and then we note the lifting of the back foot, heel first and later the rest of it as the weight of the body comes fully onto the forward foot, and the cycle continues: moving, placing, shifting—lifting, moving, placing, shifting—lifting, moving, placing, shifting.…

For each aspect of the walking, we can be in touch with the full spectrum of sensations in the body associated with walking: the lifting of the heel of the back foot, the swing of the leg as it moves forward, the placing of the heel on the ground or floor, the shifting of the weight squarely onto the forward foot, and with the seamless integration of all these elements, the continuity of walking, if ever so slowly. We can coordinate these various aspects of the walking cycle with the breath, or simply observe how the breath moves as the body moves. Of course, that will depend in large measure on how slowly or quickly you are walking. In the slow walking, we take small steps. It is just regular walking, only slow. No need to exaggerate or stylize the movements of walking, even if the impulse arises. We are just talking about ordinary walking, only slower, only mindful.

One way to play with the breath if you would like to experiment with coordinating the breath and the step cycle is to breathe in as the back heel comes up, and then breathe out without moving anything else; we pause during this out-breath. Then, on the next in-breath, the back foot lifts completely and swings forward. On the out-breath, we bring the heel of that foot, now the forward foot, down to make contact. On the next in-breath, as the back heel comes up, the forward foot goes all the way down flat and the weight shifts onto that foot. On the out-breath, we pause again. On the next in-breath, we bring the back foot forward, and so we continue, moment by moment, breath by breath, and step by step. If that is too constrained, contrived, or taxing for you, you can just let the breath move as it will.

Then there are your hands. What to do with them? How about just being aware of them? You can let your arms dangle straight down, or you can hold your hands behind your back, or in front of you, either down low or up nearer the chest. Let them find a way to be at rest, and at peace, and a part of the whole of the body, and of the experience of the body walking.

Keep in mind that all these instructions are merely scaffolding, and there are a number of different methods you could experiment with in walking meditation. Ultimately, as with all the other formal practices, there is no single right way, and you can experiment with what feels most effective for you in terms of being with walking. The practice is simply walking and knowing that you are walking, and feeling, discerning, knowing non-conceptually and directly what the body walking actually is. In other words, being here for the walking, in the walking, being with every step, and not getting out ahead of yourself.

As they like to say in the Zen tradition, when walking, just walk. That is a lot easier said than done, just as it is for sitting. For again, you will find, we all find, that the mind will do what it will and thus, the body could be walking with the mind totally preoccupied with something else. The challenge in mindful walking is to keep mind and body together in the present moment with just what is happening. What is happening, as in all moments, is extremely complex. But in walking, we attempt to keep the sensations associated with walking center stage in the field of awareness, and keep reestablishing contact with them when our mind is carried off someplace else. In this way, mindful walking is no different from any other mindfulness practice, and the field of awareness can be collimated or expanded to whatever degree you care to, from noting the sensations in the feet from moment to moment to choiceless awareness of the vast spaciousness of the nowscape, even as you are walking.

We haven't come to the formal instructions for it yet, but in quick preview, you can even practice lovingkindness while walking, invoking step by step the people you wish to include in the field of lovingkindness. With each step, you can invoke one person over and over again. Or you might invoke a sequence of people, one for each step, and then cycle through the sequence: May this person be happy; may that person be happy. May this person be free from harm; may that person be free from harm. You will get the idea after going over that chapter. This works best if you are walking slowly and mindfully, fully in your body.

*

If you look for the truth outside yourself,
It gets farther and farther away.
Today, walking alone,

I meet him everywhere I step.
He is the same as me.
Yet I am not him.
Only if you understand this way
Will you merge with the way things are.

TUNG-SHAN (807–869)

YOGA

This is not the place to go into the details of yoga practice. Suffice it to say that yoga is one of the great gifts on the planet, and availing yourself of it and bringing mindfulness to your body and mind through the gateways of yoga asanas and the flowing sequences of various postures can be extraordinarily uplifting, rejuvenating, invigorating, illuminating, transporting, and just plain relaxing. You can think of yoga as a full-bodied, three-hundred-and-sixty-degree musculo-skeletal conditioning that naturally leads to greater strength, balance, and flexibility as you practice. It is a profound meditation practice in its own right, especially when practiced mindfully. It develops strength, balance, and flexibility of mind even as it is developing those same capacities at the level of the body. It is also a great doorway into stillness, into the rich complexity of the body and its potential for healing, and, as with any other meditative practice, a perfect platform for choiceless awareness. Many of our patients in the MBSR Clinic find yoga to be an extremely congenial and powerful form of mindfulness practice.

While this is not the place to go into it in detail, for the purposes of whetting our interest and broadening our understanding, it might be useful to point out that sitting is a yoga posture (indeed, there are many sitting postures in yoga), standing is a yoga posture (called the mountain), and as we have already seen, lying down is a yoga posture (the corpse pose). And so is virtually every other posture the body can conjure up, especially if it is entered into with awareness. In hatha yoga, there are said to be over 84,000 primary postures, and with at least ten possible variations for each one, that makes for over 840,000 yoga postures, which means a virtually infinite number of ways of combining and sequencing them. So there is always plenty of room for exploration and innovation. What is more, mindful breathing is a key part of yoga practice. How we breathe while moving into and maintaining various postures, the qualities and depth of the breath in different configurations of the body, and most importantly, the quality of our awareness of the breath in the body and of what the senses and the mind are up to from moment to moment are of central and critical importance in practicing yoga mindfully.

In yoga, the postures themselves are of secondary importance compared to the attitude we bring to the practice in terms of both presence of mind and openness of heart. Of course, out of the 84,000 primary yoga postures, there are a relatively small number of basic sequences and practices, and these can be learned from a broad range of superb teachers who can be found in the many different yoga schools, programs, and retreat centers within the various yoga traditions, where you can not only learn the practices but practice regularly with others. The flowering of yoga in the West is one of the marks of the yearning for and the movement toward a greater consciousness of mind and body, and of a greater commitment to true well-being and health across the life span on the part of millions of people, young and old alike. The same is true for tai chi and chi gung.

Mindful hatha yoga has been an intimate part of MBSR since the beginning. It is also an important component of the Dr. Dean Ornish Heart Healthy Lifestyle Program, which has been shown to reverse heart disease, and of the Commonweal Cancer Help Program developed by Rachel Remen and Michael Lerner. Mindful yoga can be practiced extremely gently and slowly, and can be entered into by virtually anybody in some form or other, even if you are suffering from chronic pain, have a long-standing injury, or have been sedentary for decades. You can even practice yoga lying in bed, or in a wheelchair. You can also practice it aerobically. There are many different schools of yoga that present it in different ways, depending on their particular lineage. But again, in essence, yoga is universal, and the postures are a reflection of the extraordinary range of the human body's capacity for movement, balance, and stillness.

Our patients are encouraged to visualize themselves doing postures they are unable to assume because of an injury or chronic pain. Curiously, that too can have its effects, perhaps by priming the nervous system and musculature for future attempts to practice, once the inflammation of certain regions has been reduced, as well as by increasing concentration, confidence, and intentionality just by imagining yourself doing it. Engaging gently in a few postures to whatever degree you can manage at first, with whatever parts of the body can be recruited for the purpose, begins the process of reducing disuse atrophy, speeding recovery, and mobilizing different regions of the body for greater activity. With ongoing practice, this frequently results in increased range of motion for many joints and thus greater flexibility—an increased number of degrees of freedom in moving the body, in addition to greater strength and balance.

Just as it is important to practice formal sitting or lying down meditation on a regular basis, so it is valuable to work with your body by practicing yoga in this way on a regular, even daily basis. There is nothing quite so wonderful as getting your body down on the floor on a yoga mat or well-padded carpet and working with it gently and systematically and above all, mindfully, using the various asanas and sequences of postures to gradually re-inhabit your body with awareness and explore its ever-changing boundaries, limits, and capabilities in the present moment. Over days, weeks, months, and years, you are likely to find your body and your mind changing in remarkable ways no matter what your age, and no matter what the condition of your body when you start. The secret is to be gentle and always work this side of your limits in any given moment. That way, you reduce the likelihood of overstretching or straining muscles, ligaments, and joints, and give your body the greatest opportunity to grow into itself, usually well beyond its apparent limitations. Again, there is no end to it, and even tiny efforts are sufficient and important. As always, "this is it," so the inhabiting is always happening here and now. The journey itself continues to be the destination, even if you are setting progressive goals for yourself to motivate you and mobilize your energies. At the same time, there is also no journey and no destination. Only this moment.

The body, if attended to in this way, will wind up teaching you what you need to know to best insure its well-being moment by moment. It is feelable, knowable right in this moment if we let go into the experience with no expectations. If the body gets stronger and healthier over time, so much the better. Moreover, chances are the yoga will complement and help refine and deepen not only your sitting practice, but also and most importantly, your cultivation of embodied mindfulness in everyday life—the real meditation practice and the real yoga practice when all is said and done.

Through the practice of mindful yoga, we can expand and deepen our sense of what it means to *inhabit* the body and develop a richer and more nuanced sense of the lived body in the lived moment. In fact, the deep meaning of the word "rehabilitation" actually means to learn to live inside again (from the French *habiter*, which means to dwell, to inhabit). The Indo-European root is *ghabe*, meaning giving and receiving.

Now, what on earth does giving and receiving have to do with inhabiting the body? Well, when taking up residence in a new apartment or house, don't we in a sense give ourselves over to the new space, its features and qualities, where the rooms are located, the flow patterns of moving through it, how the sunlight falls in different rooms at different times of the day, where the doors and the windows are, and what the energy flow in the space is like? And doesn't the space, over time, if we are receptive to it, give back to us a sense of what should go where, how best to inhabit it, what kinds of renovations might in time improve its usefulness for us? We can't know all of this by jumping to conclusions too early, on the day we first see it, or even on the day we move in. We have to slowly let the space reveal itself to us, and that can only happen if we are willing to "receive" it. This kind of sensitivity is a form of wisdom. In China, it is called *feng shui,* and there is an entire art and science to it.

Similarly, when the body is in need of rehabilitation, especially in the aftermath of an illness or injury, or if suffering from a chronic disease or pain condition, or after simply neglecting the body for a significant stretch of time, we give ourselves over to the entire field of the body, to the bodyscape as we find it. We do this in large measure by feeling it moment by moment, by sensing it, by exploring it through the mind and through mindful, gentle moving. In this way, if we attend carefully, the body gives back to us, informs us, lets us know how it is and what its limits and its needs are in this moment. The reciprocity of *relationality* between the felt body and our lived experience of it facilitates the actual day-to-day, moment-by-moment learning to live inside again. Whose body and whose life does not require and even long for at one time or other such restoration, such rehabilitation? And do we have to wait until we are injured or suffering from an illness before we begin?

The degree to which the body will respond is unknown, always uncertain, never to be assumed or taken for granted. But it loves the process. It loves the care and mindful attention. And…it responds in ways hard to imagine, and sometimes, even hard to believe.

In *The Healing Power of Mindfulness*, we will encounter an extreme and extremely remarkable example of deep rehabilitation in the case of the actor, the late Christopher Reeve, who was paralyzed with a spinal cord injury after being thrown from a horse. But the same principles of healing and recovery of function underlie the practice for anyone who is doing yoga mindfully or bringing mindfulness to the body exercising, and particularly, for all of the MBSR participants who engage in mindful yoga as part of their own rehabilitation and healing, each working at his or her own level in any and every moment.

The rehabilitation of the body—in the sense of fully inhabiting it and cultivating intimacy with it as it is, however it is—is a universal attribute of mindfulness practice in general as well as of mindful yoga in particular. And since ultimately it is of limited value to speak of the body as separate from the mind, or of mind separated from body, we are inevitably talking about the rehabilitation of our whole being, and the rediscovery of our intrinsic wholeness moment by moment, step by step, and breath by breath starting, as always, from where we are now.

Just Knowing

As we have been seeing, within any posture for formally practicing mindfulness meditation—lying down, sitting, standing, or even while walking or doing yoga—you can, if you care to, intentionally and specifically feature the thinking process itself in the field of awareness, watching your thoughts as discrete events arising and passing away like clouds in the sky.

This can be a great spectator sport, at least until the "spectator" aspect that accompanies the inevitable instructional scaffolding for following a particular method falls away on its own, as it will over time. By observing the very process of thinking itself, you get to see how such tiny and short-lived "events" within the mind, which have no substantial existence and which are often completely illusory or highly inaccurate or irrelevant, can nevertheless be so consequential. You get to see how dramatically—as when we get really angry—they can affect our states of mind and body, influence our decisions with potentially devastating downstream consequences for ourselves and others, and prevent us from seeing and being present with things as they actually are in any given moment. The practice of watching your thoughts from moment to moment—especially if you stop thinking of them as "yours"— can be profoundly illuminating and liberating. It can also be quite humbling, since it is so easy for us to get completely caught up in the thought stream.

One way to practice mindfulness of thinking, whatever body posture you adopt, is to just give yourself over to watching and sensing the arising of individual thoughts as if they were bubbles coming off the bottom of a pot of water as it comes to boiling, or the gurglings of a mountain stream passing over and around rocks in a streambed.

Another image that may be helpful in refining this practice is to think of watching your thoughts as if you were turning off the sound on your television and then observing what is actually going on on the screen, without captions of course. The content immediately loses a lot of its power, and you see everything differently because you are not so sucked in, so caught up and absorbed in the content, the commentary, the emotion, the drama. There is more of a chance to see your thoughts as events in the field of awareness, like clouds in the sky, or writing on water—and ultimately, for pure seeing, pure knowing.

As we have noted many times already, our thoughts seem to come in strings or chains or like cars down a street. They proliferate one out of another, sometimes obviously connected, in other moments bizarrely random or disconnected. Sometimes the stream of thoughts is a mere trickle. At other times, it is a roaring torrent, a cascading waterfall. The challenge is always the same... to see individual thoughts *as thoughts*, and not get caught by their content or emotional charge, even as we perceive all that as well. In this way, our thoughts can be recognized and known as mere occurrences, discrete events in the field of awareness. We can know them *as thoughts* as they arise, as they linger, and as they fade away—usually into the next thought in an unending stream. Another challenge we could play with is to see or feel *the spaces* between those thoughts, and let the awareness rest in the spaces as well as in the embrace of the thought events themselves.

In this way, we intentionally take up residency in awareness itself. We rest in awareness, in the field of non-conceptual knowing that immediately apprehends, like a mirror, any disturbance within itself, any appearance of a thought forming, a droplet, a secretion, an eddy, a nucleation of an idea, an opinion, a judgment, a bubble, a longing that might arise within the stream, within the torrent. The thought is directly and immediately seen and known. Its content is seen and known. Its emotional charge is seen and known.

And that is all. We don't move to pursue it or suppress it, hold on to it or push it away. It is merely seen and known, recognized, if you will, and thereby "touched" by awareness itself, by an instantaneous registering of it as a thought. And in that touching, in that knowing, in that seeing, the thought, like a soap bubble that we touch with a finger, goes poof, dissipates, dissolves, evaporates instantly. As we noted before, it could be said, as the Tibetans do, that in that moment of recognition, it self-liberates. It merely arises and passes away in the spaciousness of the field of awareness itself, without our effort, without our intention for it to do so, just like waves on the ocean rise up for a brief moment, and then fall back into the ocean itself, thus losing their identity, their momentary relative self-hood, returning to their undifferentiated water-nature. We have done nothing, other than desist from feeding the thought in any way, which would only make it proliferate into another thought, another wave, another bubble.

As a consequence, we become increasingly familiar with thoughts as thoughts, as momentary mind events rather than the truth of anything. We come to see our narratives as just that, constructed or fabricated, not necessarily true or true enough. We come to see that we can, out of pure being, out of pure non-doing and non-reaction, rest in our being without getting caught so frequently by our thoughts and feelings. Our speech and our actions, even the way we are in our body and the expressions on our face are no longer so tightly coupled to our thoughts. Because we are seeing more clearly from moment to moment, we can let go of more and more unwise, reactive, self-absorbed, aggressive, or fearful impulses, even as they are letting go of us and washing through us because of our knowing. So there is a mutual freeing here when we see and know that our thoughts are just thoughts, not the truth of things, and certainly not accurate representations of who we are. In being seen and known, they cannot but self-liberate, and we are, in that moment, liberated from them.

In the daily conduct of our lives, as well as during formal meditation practice, it is extremely helpful to know that we are not our thoughts (including our ideas and opinions and even strongly held views) and that they are not necessarily true, or only true to a degree, and often not so helpful anyway. It is when we don't even know thoughts as thoughts, when there is no awareness of the stream of thought itself and the individual bubbles and currents and whirlpools of thought within the stream, that we have no way to reliably free ourselves from their incredibly powerful and persistent but often deluded hold over us.

JUST HEARING

As we have noted any number of times now, sounds and the spaces between sounds never stop arriving at our ears. As we sit or lie someplace in meditation, if we are giving ourselves over to some form of practice right in this moment, if you are open to it, we can intentionally attend to hearing…just hearing what is here to be heard in this moment, nothing more. I invite you to play with it for a few moments, right now.

Hearing what is here to be heard means we have nothing to do. The sounds are already coming to our ears. They are always arriving. Our challenge is, can we hear them? Can we be with them moment by moment: sounds and the spaces between sounds met with awareness, just as we have been doing with thoughts and the spaces between them—without liking or disliking, preferring or rejecting, without judging or evaluating, cataloguing or savoring? Of course, you can intentionally do this with music, which is itself a rich and wonderful practice, but the challenge here is to practice with whatever sounds are already presenting themselves, often not always so pleasant, unless you are in pristine nature. But for this practice, it doesn't matter, because we are practicing non-attachment to pleasant or unpleasant. We are practicing just hearing.

We could call it being with hearing. See if you can be here in the pure awareness of hearing. Of course, in any given moment there may very well be thoughts arising about what you are hearing, and feelings that accompany the thoughts, a range of emotions with a range of strengths and positive or negative charges, depending on what the sounds evoke, perhaps memories, perhaps fantasies, perhaps nothing. In all cases, over and over again if necessary—and it will be necessary—letting whatever is not sound be in the wings and feature pure hearing center stage in the field of awareness, until perhaps there is no longer any center, any stage, or any wings. And perhaps there is no longer any "you" who "has" to be listening, and nothing to be listened for or to. There is, instead, just hearing, before and underneath everything else, just the bare experience of hearing and the non-conceptual awareness of hearing that mindfulness already is.

As you give yourself over to hearing in this way, you are invited to rest in the bare experiencing of it moment by moment, and to come back to it over and over again when you are carried off by whatever activity is happening "offstage" and you finally notice it. Because as soon as you are carried off, there is thinking, and then there is the need for refocusing, for a bit of scaffolding and a method to reposition or redirect your attention. All of a sudden, there is a "you" again, and a stage, and, as well, the possibility to return to hearing, pure and simple. In such moments, reformulating the intention to pay attention and to sustain attention, to surrender over and over, again and again to the hearing that is always happening without your having to do anything or exert yourself at all. In fact, in such moments, you can let go of yourself completely, opening once again to sounds and the spaces between sounds, and to the silence lying inside and underneath all sound. We are allowing sound and awareness to be co-extensive, so that every sound or moment of silence itself is immediately met, immediately known, without thinking, for just what it is. For that is what the essence of mind, what we have been calling "original mind," does...it knows non-conceptually. It already knows, without thinking, before thinking even arises.

Dwelling in hearing, becoming hearing, merging with hearing, until—and this may be only for brief moments at first—there is no hearer and nothing being listened for or to, nothing but hearing, hearing, hearing...a purity of awareness without center or periphery, without subject or object, that can be visited and touched over and over, sustaining itself as your familiarity with the practice deepens.

Just Breathing

Just as sounds never stop arriving at our ears, so the breath never stops arising and completing itself as long as we are alive. In every moment of now, we are always somewhere in the breath cycle of in or out or in the brief pauses between them. So, when practicing either sitting or lying down, standing, walking, or doing yoga, the invitation is to give yourself over to the sensations throughout the body that are associated with breathing, sensations that we seldom recognize or attend to or care about, unless of course we are choking or drowning, or we have a bad cold, so much do we take breathing for granted and tune it out.

Now, in cultivating mindfulness of breathing, we are purposefully tuning in to these breath sensations, and we are doing so gently, with a lightness of touch, allowing our attention to approach the breath, as we have said before, as if we were coming upon a shy animal sunning itself on a tree stump in a forest clearing—with that kind of gentleness and interest, not so much in stealth as in wonder.

Or, to invoke another image, allowing your attention to alight on the breath as a leaf might flutter down onto the surface of a pond, and then resting here, riding on the waves of the breath, so to speak, as it moves into the body and as it exits the body. Seeing if you can be in touch with the full duration of each breath coming in, in touch with the full duration of each breath going out, and with the pauses at the top and the bottom, the apex and trough, the apogee and perigee of each full swing of one breath. You are not so much *thinking* about the breath or the breath sensations. Rather, you are *feeling* the breath sensations as vividly and intimately as possible as you ride on the waves of the breath like a leaf, or as if you were floating on a rubber raft on some gently lapping waves on the ocean or a lake. In this way, you are giving yourself over completely to the breath sensations, moment by moment by moment.

> *Only trust.*
> *Don't the leaves flutter down*
> *just like this?*

In giving yourself over to breathing, in aiming and sustaining your attention moment by moment, you invite the sense of an observer observing the breath to dissolve into just breathing. The subject (you) and the object (the breath, or even "my breath") dissolve into breath*ing*, pure and simple, and into an awareness that needs no "you" to generate it, that already knows breathing as it is unfolding, beyond thinking, underneath thinking, before thinking, just as we saw for hearing. Sitting here breathing, there is just this moment, just this breath, just this non-conceptual knowing. The whole body is breathing, the skin, the bones, all of it, inside and out, and being breathed as much as breathing, beyond any thoughts we may have about it. Resting here, we are the breathing, we are the knowing, moment by moment, if there are still moments, breath by breath if there are still breaths... tasting the breath, smelling the breath, drinking in the breath, allowing yourself to be breathed, to be touched by the air, caressed by the air, to merge with the air in the lungs, across the skin, everywhere the air, everywhere the breath in the body, everywhere the knowing, and nowhere too. And of course, as with all the other practices, we come back over and over again to an awareness of breathing when the mind wanders into thought, into memory or anticipation, into stories of one kind or another, even stories about how you are meditating and being completely one with the breath, or that there is no "you" anymore.

And although it is natural that we say that "I am breathing" and that it is "my" breath, it is also helpful to keep in mind that the fact of the matter is that if it were up to us to keep the breathing going, we would have died long ago. We are too distractible and unreliable to be in charge of the breathing process. We get caught up in a thought, or get a text or an e-mail and forget about keeping the breathing going and...whoops, we are dead. So whoever *you* think you are, your very biology doesn't allow "you" anywhere near the circuitry of the brainstem, the phrenic nerve, and the diaphragm that together keep you breathing, even during sleep. It would be much more accurate to say that you are being breathed rather than claiming that you are breathing. That would be much less self-centered. Such an orientation also reminds us of the gift and mystery behind who we think we are, and reminds us that we are much bigger than the narratives we create about our experiences and about who and what we are.

Lovingkindness Meditation

For a long time, even though it was in there, I felt somewhat ambivalent about including lovingkindness as a meditation practice in its own right within the MBSR curriculum. There were several reasons. First, I felt that in some fundamental way, all meditation practices, when seen as radical acts of sanity and love, are also acts of lovingkindness. After all, the emphasis we place on mindfulness as an affectionate, openhearted attention, coupled with the welcoming and entertaining of all the visitors to the guesthouse, is itself a gesture of great hospitality and kindness toward oneself. What is more, the suggestion that just sitting with yourself is a radical act of love captured, I felt, the essence of lovingkindness and beneath it, the overriding ethical spirit and intention of the practice to at least do no harm. Moreover, the entire culture of MBSR has always attempted to ground itself in embodied lovingkindness and an honoring of Hippocratic principles. So to my mind, nothing needed to be said explicitly. Better to be loving and kind, as best we could be in all aspects of our work with our patients and leave it at that.

But my biggest reservation concerning teaching lovingkindness as a formal meditation practice was that it might be confusing for people who were in the early stages of being introduced for the first time to the attitude and practice of non-doing and non-striving that underlie all the meditation practices we have touched on so far that constitute the core of MBSR. I did not want it to undermine that orientation of direct, moment-to-moment, non-reactive, non-judgmental attending that is so unusual for us as Americans to even consider adopting, and that can be so deeply transformative and liberating if we take it seriously and, through our own wise efforts and discipline, fashion it into a way of being.

The reason for my hesitation was that in the instructions for lovingkindness meditation, there is an inevitable sense that you are being invited to engage in *doing something*, namely invoking particular feelings and thoughts and generating desirable states of mind and heart. This feels very different from and often outright contradictory to simply *observing* whatever is naturally arising in experience without recruiting one's thoughts or feelings to any particular end other than awareness itself. I didn't want to wind up confusing people about the core practice and attitude of non-doing, since it is the foundation of non-dual mindfulness practice, of the wisdom and compassion that arise naturally from it, and of everything we teach in MBSR.

I also didn't want to confuse people simply by throwing too many new things at them in a short period of time. After all, meditation is a huge and elaborate edifice, when you consider all the various practices available in even one tradition. Cultivating and refining intimacy with even a small part of it is nothing short of a lifetime engagement. It is impossible to enter into a building through all its various doors at once, and folly just to keep going in and out through them. If you do, you will never wind up spending any time inside.

Without papering over these differences, it still felt that people in the MBSR Clinic should have at least a taste of formal lovingkindness practice because of its potential to touch our hearts in such deep ways and contribute to a strengthening of love and kindness in the world. Moreover, while everything I have said is true at face value, on a deeper level, the instructions for loving-kindness only *appear* to be making something happen. Under-neath, they are simply revealing feelings we actually already have but that are usually so buried that they need continual invitation to emerge. Ultimately, we are talking about the human heart as it is, knowing and touching itself as it is. That knowing and that touching are virtually boundless. And so, although for pedagogical and practical reasons we do not include training in formal loving-kindness meditation on a par with the training in formal sitting and lying down meditations in MBSR unless particular individual or group circumstances warrant it, we do introduce people to it as a guided meditation during the all-day silent retreat in the sixth week of the program.

Lovingkindness, or *metta* in the Pali language, is one of four foundational practices taught by the Buddha, known collectively as the divine or heavenly abodes. The four are lovingkindness, com-passion, sympathetic joy, and equanimity. All of these are rigor-ous meditation practices in their own right, used for the most part to cultivate *samadhi* or one-pointed concentrated attention, out of which the powers of the evoked qualities emerge, transfiguring the heart. But the essence of all these practices is contained and acces-sible within all the mindfulness practices we have already touched on. Even so, just naming these qualities of heart and making their role explicit in our practice may help us to recognize them when they arise spontaneously during mindfulness practice, as well as to help us incline the heart and mind in their direction more fre-quently, especially in difficult times. In fact, these practices can sometimes serve as a necessary and skillful antidote to mind states such as ferocious anger, which may at the time of their arising be simply too strong to attend to via direct observation unless one's practice is fairly well-developed. At such times, formal lovingkindness practice can function to soften one's relationship to such overwhelmingly afflictive mind states so that we can avoid succumbing completely to their energies. It also makes such mind states more approachable and less intractable. However, as we have seen, with concerted and sustained practice, mindfulness itself can embrace any mind state, however afflictive or toxic, and in the seeing of it and the knowing of it within the openhearted, non-reactive, non-judgmental embrace of awareness, we can see directly into the nature of the anger or grief or whatever it is, and in the seeing, in the embracing of it, in the knowing of it, that mind state attenuates, weakens, evaporates, very much like touching a soap bubble or like writing on water. What emerges in such moments is nothing less than lovingkindness itself, arising naturally from extended silence, without any invitation, because it is never not already here.

In teaching or practicing formal lovingkindness meditation, I sometimes include imagery, emphasizing the direct feeling of lovingkindness rather than rely solely on the traditional phrases associated with evoking it. What follows is a guided lovingkindness meditation you might explore whenever you care to—even now.

In a sitting posture or lying down, or standing, whenever you are ready, bringing your awareness to the breath and the body as a whole breathing. Resting here for a period of time, establishing a relatively stable platform of moment-to-moment awareness, riding on the waves of the breath.

When you feel comfortable resting within the natural flowing of your breathing, picturing in your mind's eye someone in your life who loves you or loved you totally and unconditionally. Recalling the *feeling* of the love and kindness they accorded you, the whole aura of their love for you. Breathing with these feelings, bathing in them, resting in their total acceptance and embracing of you just as you are or were. Noticing that you are loved and accepted without having to be different, without having to be worthy of their love, without having to be particularly deserving. In fact, you may not feel particularly worthy or deserving. That does not matter. In fact, it is irrelevant. The relevant fact is that you were or are loved wholeheartedly. Their love is or was for you just as you are, for who you are now, already, and perhaps always have been. It is truly unconditional.

Allowing your whole being to bask in these feelings right now, to be cradled in them, to be rocked moment by moment by the rhythmic swing of your own heartbeat, and in the flowing cadences of your own breathing, embraced by and bathing in this field of benevolence, this field of lovingkindness, in the total acceptance of who you are or were. And resting here in this feeling for as long as you like, or for as long as it lasts.

And if you are unable to bring to mind or conjure up such a person from memory, as is true for so many of us, then seeing if you can *imagine* someone treating you in that way. That works fine as well.

Now, whenever you feel ready, seeing if you can become *the source* as well as the receiver of these same feelings, in other words, taking on these very same loving feelings for yourself as if they were your own rather than those of another. Linger with the rhythmic beating of your own heart, inviting into your own heart these feelings of love and acceptance and kindness for yourself, beyond judgment of any kind, just basking in feelings of loving-kindness akin to the embrace of a mother for her child, where you are simultaneously both the mother and the child. Resting here in these feelings as best you can from moment to moment, breath by breath, bathing in your own kind regard and acceptance of yourself as you are. Letting this feeling be self-sustaining, natural, in no way forced or coerced. Even tiny tastes of it are balm and succor for all the negativity and self-criticism and self-loathing that can lie beneath the surface of our psyches.

In resting here in this field of lovingkindness, this embrace of lovingkindness, you may find it useful to whisper to yourself inwardly the following phrases, or hear them being whispered to you by the wind, by the air, by the breath, by the world:

May I be safe and protected and free from inner and
    outer harm
May I be happy and contented
May I be healthy and whole to whatever degree possible
May I experience ease of well-being...

At first, it may feel artificial to be saying such things to yourself, or even thinking them. After all, who is this "I" who is wishing this? And who is the "I" who is receiving these wishes? Ultimately, both vanish into the *feeling* of being safe and free from harm in this moment; into the *feeling* of being contented and happy in this moment; the *feeling* of being whole in this moment, since you already are whole; the *feeling* of resting in ease of well-being, far from the dis-ease and fragmentation we endure so much of the time. This feeling is the essence of lovingkindness.

But, you might object, if this is a selfless practice, why am I focusing on myself, on my own feelings of safety and well-being, on my own happiness? One response: because you are not separate from the universe that gave rise to you, and so are as worthy a receiver of lovingkindness as anything else or anyone else. Your lovingkindness cannot be either loving or kind if it does not include yourself, can it? But at the same time, you don't need to worry. It is not limited to yourself because the field of lovingkindness is limitless. If you like, you can think of the lovingkindness practice as described up to this point as merely (but importantly) tuning your instrument before you play it out in the world. In this case, tuning the instrument is itself a huge act of love and kindness and wisdom in and of itself, not merely a means to an end.

The practice continues...

Once you have established a fairly stable field of lovingkindness around yourself—and it may feel different every time—and once you have lingered for a time in the feeling of being held and cradled and rocked in its embrace, you can intentionally expand the field of your own heart just as we have been learning to expand the field of awareness in the mindfulness practice. We can experiment with expanding the field of lovingkindness around our own heart and our own being, inviting other beings, either singly or *en masse*, into this growing embrace. This is not always so easy to do, and so it is helpful to start with one person for whom you naturally harbor feelings of lovingkindness.

So whenever you are ready to try it, in your mind's eye and in your heart, evoking the feeling or image of an individual for whom you have great affection, someone you are very close to emotionally, someone you can truly say you love. Can you hold this person in your heart, with the same quality of lovingkindness that you have been directing toward yourself? Whether it is a child or a parent, a brother or a sister, a grandparent or other relative near or distant, a close friend or a cherished neighbor, singly or together, breathing with them in your heart, holding them in your heart, imaging them in your heart as best you can (although none of it needs to be very vivid for it to be effective), wishing them well:

> May she, he, they be safe and protected and free from inner and outer harm
> May she, he, they be happy and contented
> May she, he, they be healthy and whole to whatever degree possible
> May she, he, they experience ease of well-being...

Lingering moment by moment in this feeling of lovingkindness within your own heart, with these words or others as you voice them silently to yourself. And lingering even more with the feeling behind the words, repeating them over and over again silently to yourself, not mechanically, but mindfully, with full awareness, knowing what you are saying, feeling the intention behind the feeling, the intention and feeling behind each phrase, and how it is expressing itself in your body, in your heart in this moment.

From here, you can invite into the field of your own loving heart those who you do not know so well, either singly or together, those for whom your relationship may be a lot more neutral, or even people you don't know at all, or who you have only heard of secondhand, friends of your friends, for instance. And again, to whatever degree you care to, cradling him, her, or them in your heart, wishing them well:

> May she, he, they be safe and protected and free from inner and outer harm
> May she, he, they be happy and contented
> May she, he, they be healthy and whole to whatever degree possible
> May she, he, they experience ease of well-being...

From here, you can expand the field of awareness to include one or more individuals who may be problematic for you in one way or another, with whom perhaps you share a difficult past, who may have harmed you in one way or another, who, for whatever reason, you consider to be more of an adversary or an obstacle than a friend. This does not mean that you are being asked to forgive them for what they may have done to hurt you or to cause you or others harm. You are simply recognizing that they too are human beings, that they too have aspirations, that they too suffer from dis-ease and perhaps disease, that they too desire to be happy and safe. So, as best you can, and only to the degree that you feel ready for it or at least open to experimenting with it, you put your toe in the water ever so cautiously, with eyes wide open, extending lov-ingkindness to them as well, while still recognizing and honoring all the difficulties and problems lying between you:

> May she, he, they be safe and protected and free from inner and outer harm
> May she, he, they be happy and contented
> May she, he, they be healthy and whole to whatever degree possible
> May she, he, they experience ease of well-being...

To pause for a moment, you can see where this is going. Just as with the cultivation of mindfulness, where we can focus on one primary object of attention or expand the field to include a range of objects to attend to, so in the lovingkindness practice, we can linger for days, weeks, months, or years at differing levels of the practice, all of which are valid, and all of which, ultimately, include each other, because after all, it is your own heart which is softening and becoming more inclusive. So if you wish to cultivate lovingkindness and direct it only toward yourself during a particular sitting, or for many many sittings, that is perfectly fine. Or if you care to direct lovingkindness only toward those you know and love, or even one person over and over again, that is just fine too.

But over time, it is likely—since your own capacity for loving, whether you know it or not, is infinite (that is simply the nature of love, it is limitless and therefore in infinite supply)—that you will find yourself naturally drawn to invite more and more beings into the field of lovingkindness radiating from you in all directions, inwardly and outwardly—even insects, even birds, even mice, even snakes or toads.

Or you may find that at times they just slip in unbidden. This is interesting to note. If you are not consciously inviting them in, how come they are showing up anyway? And how are they getting in? Hmmm. Maybe your heart is bigger and wiser than you think.

In the spirit of the boundlessness of the heart and of love, we can expand the field of lovingkindness to include our neighbors and neighborhood, our community, our state, our country, the entire world. You can include your pets, all animal life, all plant life, all life, the entire biosphere, all sentient beings. You can also get very specific, and include specific people you don't know, even political leaders, in the field of your lovingkindness, difficult as that may be if you differ strongly with them and find yourself judging them harshly and even doubting their basic humanity. All the more reason for including them. Being human, they too are worthy of lovingkindness, and perhaps will respond to it by softening in ways your mind cannot possibly imagine. And perhaps the same goes for you as well.

You can also, if you care to, specifically include in the field of lovingkindness all those less fortunate than yourself, who are exploited at work or at home, who are victims of poverty or racism or "othering," who are refugees from genocide, those who are imprisoned unjustly, as so many are, those who are at the mercy of or fleeing from endemic corruption, often legalized, those who have been traumatized, brutalized, or violated in any way. You can include all those who are presently hospitalized or sick or dying, all those who are caught up in chaos, who are living in fear, who are suffering in any way, shape, or form. Whatever brought them to this point in their lives, just as we do, they too want to experience ease of well-being rather than dis-ease and fragmentation and violence. Just as we do, they too want to be happy and contented, they too desire to be whole and healthy, they too desire to be safe and free from harm. In this way, we recognize how much we human beings, and all living creatures, are all united in our common aspiration to be happy and not to suffer, and so we wish them well:

> May all beings near and far be safe and protected and free
> from inner and outer harm
> May all beings near and far be happy and contented
> May all beings near and far be healthy and whole to
> whatever degree possible
> May all beings near and far experience ease of well-being…

And it need not stop here. Why not include the entire Earth in the field of lovingkindness? Why not embrace the very Earth that is our home, that is an organism in its own right, that is in a sense one body, a body that can be thrown off balance by our own actions, conscious and unconscious, in ways that create huge threats to the life it nurtures and to the intelligences embedded within all aspects of that life, animal and plant and mineral that interact so seamlessly in the natural world?

And so, we can expand the field of the loving heart, of our lovingkindness, to include the planet as a whole, and out beyond that, to the entirety of the universe in which even the sun is merely an atom and we...not even a quark.

> May our planet and the whole universe be safe and protected and free from harm
> May our planet and the whole universe be happy and contented
> May our planet and the whole universe be healthy and whole
> May our planet and the whole universe experience ease of well-being...

It may seem a little silly, even animistic, to wish for the happiness of the planet or the whole universe, but why not? In the end, whether we are talking about individual people who are problematic for us, or the entire universe, what is most important is that we incline our own heart toward inclusion rather than toward separation. In the end, whatever the consequences for others or for the planet or the universe, or any levels in between, the willingness to extend ourselves in this way, literally and metaphorically, to extend the reach of our own heart, has profound consequences for our own life, and for our own capacity to live in the world in ways that embody wisdom and compassion, lovingkindness and equanimity, and ultimately, that express the joy inherent in being alive, and the essentially boundless joy inherent in freeing ourselves in any moment from the weight of our mindless conditioning and the suffering that that conditioning engenders.

To engage in this way with the lovingkindness meditation is to recognize and nurture your own heart's essential freedom and inclusiveness, your own humanity in all its beauty, not in some magical future but here and now, with things exactly as they are in this moment. No doubt the world benefits in some small but not insignificant way and is purified from even one person's offering of lovingkindness. We could say that the relationships within the lattice structure of reality and the web of all life are slightly but not inconsequentially shifted through our momentary or increasingly sustained openness of heart, and through our willingness to let go of any rancor and ill will we might be harboring, however justified we may think it is.

At the same time, by our engagement in such a practice and our recognition and trusting in the deepest nature of our own hearts, we who have emerged out of the earth, out of the ongoing lifestream of humanity, out of the universe,* are somehow blessed and purified and made whole by the generosity of the very gesture of the lovingkindness practice in and of itself, and by its effects on our own heart that, for a moment at least, is no longer willing to harbor rancor and ill will. We who choose to practice and embody lovingkindness, formally or informally, if even just a little bit, are undisputedly its first but hardly its only beneficiaries.

*

---

* Let's not forget that the very atoms of our bodies were themselves forged in exploding supernovae and, in the case of the hydrogen, in the aftermath of the big bang itself, approximately 13.7 billion years ago, once the conditions allowed for its formation.

Before you know what kindness really is
you must lose things,
feel the future dissolve in a moment
like salt in a weakened broth
What you held in your hand,
what you counted and carefully saved,
all this must go so you know
how desolate the landscape can be
between the regions of kindness.
How you ride and ride
thinking the bus will never stop,
the passengers eating maize and chicken
will stare out the window forever.

Before you learn the tender gravity of kindness,
you must travel where the Indian in a white poncho
lies dead by the side of the road.
You must see how this could be you,
how he too was someone
who journeyed through the night with plans
and the simple breath that kept him alive.

Before you know kindness as the deepest thing inside,
you must know sorrow as the other deepest thing.
You must wake up with sorrow.
You must speak to it till your voice
catches the thread of all sorrows
and you see the size of the cloth.

Then it is only kindness that makes sense anymore,
only kindness that ties your shoes

and sends you out into the day to mail letters and purchase bread,
only kindness that raises its head
from the crowd of the world to say
It is I you have been looking for,
and then goes with you everywhere
like a shadow or a friend.

NAOMI SHIHAB NYE, "Kindness"

AM I DOING IT RIGHT?

It is only natural to ask such a question whenever we take on a new endeavor that involves progressing along a learning curve. Of course, we want to check and see if we are doing it correctly, whatever the "it" is, and what the signposts and benchmarks are along the way to let us know that indeed, we are making headway, not stewing in some backwater, or circling endlessly in some Sargasso Sea of the mind, that we are making progress, that we are getting somewhere and a desirable somewhere at that, at the very least that we are becoming more loving, more kind, more calm, more mindful, more heartful. And of course, we also want assurance and reassurance along the way that what we are feeling is what we are *supposed* to be feeling, that what is happening is what is *supposed* to be happening, that it is "normal," and not a sign of being incompetent or of heading in the wrong direction and perhaps unwittingly picking up a string of bad habits along the way.

Looking at meditation instrumentally (see *Meditation Is Not What You Think*, "Two Ways to Think about Meditation"), as a skill that develops as you work at it, wanting to know whether you are doing it right makes a lot of sense. And indeed there *are* benchmarks along the way, such as a greater sense of stability and calmness in your attention, an ability to sit longer and be more comfortable in your body, deeper insight and equanimity in the face of whatever might arise, a growing ability to meet whatever is arising in the field of awareness at the point of contact, and seeing the humor in how much we take everything so seriously, especially around our own particular identifications and attachments. You may even find yourself spontaneously experiencing feelings of lovingkindness, compassion, and joy in the good fortune of others.

Also, you may discover in yourself a desire and enthusiasm to practice more, a willingness to look more clearly and compassionately into places you habitually don't want to look at all, and perhaps more aware of how your states of mind affect other people as well as yourself. You may find yourself appreciating the spell and texture of the sensory world to a greater and greater degree. You may find yourself spontaneously more embodied, more in touch with your skin, with the carriage of the body, with a sense of the body as a whole breathing.

All these and many more benchmarks are available to you, and will be recognized if you just keep practicing, whether you like it or not, whether you feel like it or not, if you make the cultivation of mindfulness a lifetime's challenge and a lifetime's commitment. If you have the good fortune to work with a good teacher, that can be very helpful in terms of getting feedback about whether or not you are "doing it right," and for validating your experiences or making suggestions for ways to work with the myriad experiences that inevitably arise in the course of both living and practicing mindfulness.

But that said, there is another answer to the question, "Am I doing it right?" when it emerges in your mind and generates worry or doubt or confusion. And that answer comes from the non-instrumental nature of the meditation practice, the way in which meditation is not about getting anywhere else but simply being where you already are and knowing it. From this perspective, if you are resting in awareness, you are doing it right, no matter what you are experiencing, whether it is pleasant, unpleasant, or neutral. If you are bored and are aware of it, you are doing it right. If you are frightened and are aware of it, you are doing it right. If you are confused and know it, you are doing it right.

If you are depressed and know it, you are doing it right. If your thoughts never shut down and there is an awareness of that in the present moment, and you can, even for a moment be the knowing rather than being carried away in the agitation, then you are doing it right. And if you are indeed carried away by the agitation and the proliferations and fabrications and cascading of the thinking mind and there is an awareness of that, and you can be that knowing in that moment, then you are doing it right.

In fact, as long as you are being kind to yourself and not forcing anything, there is nothing that you could do or that could happen to you that cannot be a worthy part of the practice, if you are aware of it and can give yourself over to trusting and resting in awareness itself rather than be caught up perpetually in the turmoil, the agitation, the clinging, the wanting, and the rejecting of whatever is arising.

Of course, *dukkha* and delusion can become seriously compounded in any moment if, in losing awareness, you become caught up in unskillful and unhealthy actions or reactions that may flow out of your discomfort, your fear, or other afflictive mind states if you fall into identifying strongly with them without any awareness of it. When awareness gets obscured, clouded over, it is in just such moments that we might lose touch, even lose our minds, forget who we are in our fullness, and create impediments to our own well-being, to say nothing of possibly harming others, sometimes in the most egregious of ways. Even in such circumstances, however, awareness is always available! The practice never is not applicable. But it is much more skillful if we can gradually learn to recognize those arisings in the mind and in our actions that are potentially destructive and harmful and embrace them fully in awareness in the present moment, resolving to let that moment be a new beginning, a new opportunity to choose to restrain ourselves from harmful and destructive actions, to stand firm in that which we are.

Your awareness is a very big space within which to reside. It is never not an ally, a friend, a sanctuary, a refuge. And it is never not here, only sometimes veiled. But knowing it is subtle. The realm of awareness requires visiting many times, if ever so briefly, as you cultivate greater intimacy with it. Then, as we have seen, anything and everything that arises in life becomes "the curriculum," however unwanted or unpleasant. If you allow awareness to embrace your doubt, your unhappiness, your confusion, your anxiety, your pain, these mind states cease being "yours." They revert to being recognized as merely "weather patterns" in the mind and body. That dimension of "you" that already knows that you are doubting, unhappy, confused, anxious, in pain, resentful, even cruel at times, is not any of those things, and is already okay, already whole. It will never not be what and who you actually are at the most fundamental level. So if you remember non-judgmental awareness in the present moment as an option and learn to trust it, if you learn to inhabit the spaciousness of your own awareness or at least visit from time to time, then not only are you "doing it right" but there is actually no doing involved and never was, and nobody to do it. Mindfulness is not about doing, and never was. It is about being—and being awake, being the knowing, including the knowing of not knowing. Are they different?

Let's sit with that one for a moment.

Common Obstacles to Practice

The most common obstacle to formal meditation practice is not wanting to. Some part of you may think it is a good idea, but when the impulse to sit (or practice formally in some other way, say with the body scan or some mindful yoga) comes to you as a passing thought or feeling, other thoughts and feelings immediately crowd in, saying things like "Not now" or "Who has time?" or "I'd rather read or get in touch with so and so" or "It's time to eat soon," or "I have too much work right now" or "I'll do it later" or "I'll start tomorrow" or "I'll just be mindful doing what I'm doing." The mind is always generating thoughts that can divert or deflect that initial impulse to stop, and dwell for a time in the timeless, in stillness.

This is where intentionality and motivation come into the picture. After all, meditation is a discipline, and we benefit from it *as a discipline* when we metaphorically and literally take our seat whether we feel like it or not, no matter what other currents within the mind are offering up to deflect us from our primary purpose. So if you desire to cultivate and refine mindfulness in your life through formal practice, especially if it is new to you and you have not developed the discipline of a regular practice, or if the discipline of practice has dissipated for you over the years or become stale or denatured, you may be reassured to know that it is relatively easy to establish that core discipline or reestablish it. One powerful way is by committing yourself to waking up earlier than you normally would and making a sacrosanct time for yourself before any of the other doings and commitments of the day take over and swamp your intention. Imagine a time that is entirely for you, not to fill up or to do anything with, but simply to inhabit, to be in your own good company, to rest in as you become intimate with the unfolding of life and of life expressing itself moment by moment in your own body, and in your own mind and heart.

Of course, obstacles to meditation practice don't limit themselves to just making it hard for you to get started. Once on the cushion (this way of speaking is meant to include all the formal meditation practices we have been exploring and cultivating), there are so many ways that you can still be deflected from your intention to be present with the unfolding of whatever is arising.

First of all, the body can be squirmish, fidgety, seemingly inconsolably uncomfortable, plagued by tingling sensations, itches, or strong impulses to move and wiggle. This is no problem at all. These are just passing states and stages the body gets into and goes through. With some practice, when seen and recognized as mere sensation, those impulses and the sensations behind them can be held lightly and gently in awareness like any other impulses and sensations in the body, especially when they are not fed by inflamed thinking in the mind that is continually judging them, fighting with them, wanting to change them or surrender to them, or saying things to yourself such as: "You knew you weren't cut out to meditate," or "This confirms that meditation is sheer torture, a masochistic enterprise for those who don't already have enough suffering in their lives." This is, of course, sheer nonsense, all simply reactive mental noise on top of reactive body "noise."

As soon as you settle into the stillness underneath these sur-face waves of the mind and you become familiar with the topology of the inner and outer landscapes of your whole being, with the bodyscape, the mindscape, the nowscape, the airscape, the sense-scapes, these obstacles to practice tend to settle down and for the most part, abate. After a while, when they do make an appearance from time to time, they are just seen and known as various mind states and body states, as "weather patterns" coming and going in the field of awareness. There are always compelling reasons and ample excuses for not giving yourself over to being present right now. But as we rest in awareness anyway, even for a few moments, and allow ourselves to be the knowing, we soon see that just as with all other phenomena in the realm of experience, they do not endure.

That said, in the early stages of developing a mindfulness practice, if the resistance is particular strong, one suggestion is that you start with some mindful yoga first, and gradually ease yourself into stillness, either sitting or lying down or standing. I love doing yoga before sitting, or before a body scan or some other lying down practice.

When dropping in for any extended period of time, we readily see that the mind can get just as squirmy as the body, if not more so. You might easily run into impatience, agitation, impatience, agita-tion, impatience, agitation. You get the picture. These too are not a problem. They are merely habits of mind, along with the five so-called classical "hindrances" in the Buddha's teaching, which are indeed universal aspects of an untrained mind: sensual desire or greed; ill will or aversion; sloth and torpor—truly wonderful adjec-tives; restlessness, worry, and remorse; and doubt. As we watch them arise, linger, and pass away, along with the breath and whatever else we have chosen to include in the scope of our awareness, they too tend to be seen and known for what they are, merely impersonal mind states, and dissolve—that is, unless you feed them by struggling with them and wanting them to go away. They can serve as important, in fact, extremely useful objects of attention in their own right. You might even try making friends with your impatience, your agitations. The familiarization, the intimacy that develops from doing so *is* the meditation practice and leads to equanimity without having to dispel any of it. Pure awareness is beyond and independent of conditions and conditioning, and therefore free. What is more, it is always here, and always available, if you remember.

Sleepiness can also feel like an impediment to practice, as we have seen with the lying down meditations. But if you are serious about meditation, sleepiness does not present much of a problem. If you are totally sleep-deprived, you might try getting more sleep before you try to build or strengthen your meditation practice. The sleep-deprived mind tends to get a little crazy and lose perspective. This is best remedied by sleep. But if it is a matter of just congenitally falling asleep whenever you sit down to practice, then anything you do to support your practice makes sense, from throwing cold water on your face and neck before you come to the cushion, to taking a cold shower, or sitting with your eyes open, or standing, or all of the above. If you really want to wake up in your life and to your life, you will find good ways to support that intention and make it happen. If I am drowsy when I am driving late at night, and nothing else, such as loud rock and roll on the radio or fresh air is doing the trick, and simply stopping doesn't seem to be the thing to do at that particular moment, I will slap myself hard across the face, and more than once if necessary. In that context, it may actually be an act of wisdom and compassion. With meditation, as I've said before, it comes down to whether or not you are willing to practice as if your life depended on it. Because it does.

Another common obstacle to authentic practice is idealizing

your practice, setting impossible standards or goals for yourself and then making your practice into an act of will, almost an act of aggression, with little or no self-compassion and no sense of humor either. Most important is to not take ourselves too seriously. Remember that mindfulness practice is a radical act of love. That means that compassion and self-compassion lie at its root. If we cannot be gentle with and accepting of ourselves and the experiences we are having now, whatever they are, if we are always wanting some other, better experience to convince ourselves or others that we are "making progress," that we are becoming a "better person," then we probably should give up meditating. We will certainly be creating a great deal of stress and pain for ourselves, and then perhaps blaming the meditation practice for "not working" when it might be more accurate to say that we were unwilling to work with things as they are, as we found them, and accept ourselves as we are. Remember that the real curriculum is whatever arises moment by moment, and the challenge is how you will be in wise relationship to it. Remember that there is no improving on you, because you are already whole, already complete, already perfect as you are, including all the "imperfections." While striving and even forcing can sometimes give the impression of "progress" and "movement" and of "getting somewhere in one's practice," without self-acceptance and self-compassion, the energy of contraction and forcing is an unwise and unskillful motivation for exploring stillness. Even with the development of significant focus and stability and clarity of mind, wisdom can be elusive because it is not something that we *acquire*, but a way of seeing and a way of being that grows within us when the conditions are right. The soil of deep practice requires the fertilizer of deep self-acceptance and self-compassion. For this reason, gentleness is not a luxury, but a critical requirement for coming to our senses. Rigor and discipline are fine, even necessary, but harshness and striving ultimately only engender unawareness and insensitivity, and further fragmentation just when we have an opportunity to recognize that we are already OK, already whole, right in this moment.

In the end, obstacles to practice are infinite. Yet all of them, anticipated and unanticipated, turn into allies when they are embraced in awareness. They can feed our commitment to practice rather than impede it if we recognize them for what they are and allow them to simply be part of the nowscape—not good, not bad—because wonder of wonders, they already are.

*

When your eyes are tired
the world is tired also.

When your vision has gone
no part of the world can find you.

Time to go into the dark
where the night has eyes
to recognize its own.

There you can be sure
you are not beyond love.

The dark will be your womb
tonight.

The night will give you a horizon
further than you can see.

You must learn one thing.
The world was made to be free in.

Give up all the other worlds
except the one to which you belong.

Sometimes it takes darkness and the sweet
confinement of your aloneness
to learn

anything or anyone
that does not bring you alive

is too small for you.

DAVID WHYTE, "Sweet Darkness"

Supports for Your Practice

When all is said and done, the most important support for your mindfulness practice is the quality of your motivation and the degree of ardor you bring to it. No amount of outside support can substitute for that inward fire, that quiet passion for living life as if it really mattered, for knowing how easy it is to miss large swaths of it to unconsciousness and automaticity and to our deep conditioning. That is why I urge those who practice with me to practice as if their lives depended on it. Only if you know or even suspect that it actually does will you have sufficient energy to sit whether you feel like it or not, and really inhabit and make maximal use of that infinitude of timeless moments available to you in sitting—however long it is by the clock—without doing anything. Only if you know or even suspect that your life does indeed depend on your practice will you have sufficient energy and motivation to (1) wake up earlier than you normally would so you can have some uninterrupted time, a time just for yourself, a time for just being, a time outside of time; or (2) make a sacrosanct time for practice at some other hour of the day that works better for you; (3) practice on days when you have a lot going on; and (4) above all, make *your life* into the real meditation practice, so that it is not merely a matter of making a regular time for formal practice but of nurturing a willingness to bring mindfulness to any and every moment, no matter what you are doing or what is going on. Approaching practice in this way, it can feel after a while more like the practice is doing you rather than you are doing the practice. All this develops naturally over time. It takes less and less effort, and becomes more and more simply how you choose to live your life. But the ardor, the passion to engage in this radical act, so unusual for our time-pressured, driven way of life and the sea of distractions and demands we are so much a prey to and addicted to, is vital if we are to maintain and even deepen our momentum and commitment to liberation from the veil of our unawareness and the suffering it inevitably brings.

That said, there are an infinity of ways to strengthen and support that quiet passion for wakefulness and the determination to live free of our conditioning. We might begin by perceiving just how much we are in its grip, literally from moment to moment, and by taking steps, through that very perceiving and that very knowing, to disentangle ourselves from it. We can recognize each moment as a branch point, and hone our senses, our sensibility, our ability to steer around the obstacles and challenges and pitfalls that each moment inevitably provides, and thus, experience ourselves navigating, moving, flowing instinctually toward greater clarity, calmness, and non-clinging, however many bumps and obstacles present themselves along the way.

Most important is to remember that there is no one right way to practice, and that ultimately, you have to make the practice your own, or rather, let it gradually become yours by your willingness to give yourself over to it and let it become your teacher. Actually, it is life itself that becomes the teacher, and the curriculum. If you pay attention and keep your eyes open, you will see over and over again that it is an extraordinary teacher, even in the most ordinary of moments and in the simplest of occurrences. And the "classroom," so to speak, is the entire landscape of the inner and the outer worlds, the sensescapes, the mindscape, the nowscape, and everything that happens within them—everything, without exception—including the emptiness, the silence, the fullness of awareness that can and does hold it all. In this world, there are no obstacles to practice, only the appearance of obstacles.

There is no substitute for the ardor and passion you bring to your life, and to living it fully and gratefully. If you were the only person on the planet cultivating mindfulness, there would be no reason to give up, although it is admittedly a rather discouraging thought. In fact, it would be all the more reason to practice.

But one of the most powerful supports in practicing, at least I have found it to be so, is knowing that there are millions of people who are committed to mindfulness and to living a life of aware-ness, and that at any one moment on the planet, millions of them are actually sitting. So that when *you* take *your* seat, whenever that is, morning, noon, or night, you can know that you are not alone. You are "logging on" to a silent "presencing" that knows no bounds and has no center and no periphery. You are joining a very large community of like-minded human beings who share your pas-sion for wakefulness and liberation. And with every day, more and more people are coming to the practice through the thousands of avenues that are nowadays available to folks that in times past were simply not there.

As was mentioned in *Meditation Is Not What You Think* (see "Dukkha Magnets"), the Buddhist term for this community of people committed to the dharma is called "the Sangha," with a capital *S*, just as Dharma is often capitalized when it refers to the teaching of the Buddha in a Buddhist context. Originally "Sangha" referred to the community of monks and nuns who renounced the worldly life to follow the teachings of the Buddha. And that is still one very important meaning of the term. But the word has taken on a broader meaning to include everybody who is committed to a life of mindfulness and non-harming. We are all part of that sangha, with a small *s*, whether we know it or not, if we have even the slightest impulse to practice. It is not an organization that you join, it is a community that you are part of by virtue of your commitment and passion and caring. And having that connection can itself be a huge support in one's practice.

One image that appeals to me is that we are all leaves on the same tree. We each have our own unique location and view from where we find ourselves. We are each whole, and the whole tree depends on each one of us for its life, for its sustenance, and we on it. At the same time that we are whole, we are also part of this much larger whole, in fact, part of nested levels of wholeness that know no bounds.

No matter how we came to the practice, or will come to the practice, it is the case that neither you nor I made it up. Mindfulness as both a formal practice and a way of being has been handed down to us for us to experiment with, to explore, and to see for ourselves what it might have to offer—and to do so with the greatest integrity and reverence for what has been given and for the suffering and the ardor and the genius out of which it emerged. There is a lineage of women and men, stretching back for millennia, who were committed to the dharma and to wisdom and compassion in the same way that those of us who practice now are or can be if we so choose. These are William Butler Yeats's "unknown instructors" (see *Meditation Is Not What You Think*: "On Lineage and the Uses and Limitations of Scaffolding"). And as with any worthy lineage, at one time or another we will probably be filled with gratitude for their legacy and their gifts to us. Many of them left records of their experiences in many different languages and cultures, and many more didn't. But the sum total of the legacy is in our opportunity to avail ourselves of the spirit, the methods, the scaffolding, and the emptiness—in a word, the dharma—that they bequeathed to us by virtue of having come before us and having cared. This is a bequeathing of the species to the species. Its vitality has never been more vibrant, nor the need for it greater. This is part of the love affair, a wisdom transmission emanating from the evolutionary arc of humanity itself across the ages.

We are blessed to live at an extraordinary moment in which universal dharma in all its manifestations has never been more accessible. Books by respected meditation teachers and scholars are now available as never before, as are podcasts and YouTube videos. We are proffered a veritable cornucopia of opportunities to learn from great teachers in different lineages, an extraordinary abundance that is continuing to build over time. I provide a relatively short list of some of those books and organizations that have had the greatest impact on my life and the lives of my students and colleagues at the back of this book. Guided meditations in various formats available online that instruct and facilitate aspects of mindfulness practice can also be valuable if not critical resources and supports for developing and deepening your practice. They include the guided meditations I developed for MBSR and to accompany various books of mine. These are described on the last page of this book.

But when all is said and done, it still comes down to getting your rear end on the cushion. Reading can be inspirational, as can coming in contact with great teachers either in person or though podcasts, websites, and videos. Sitting with others can be hugely supportive (more on this below), but you still have to practice yourself, with your body and with your mind, and with your situation.

You can overdose on books, and the books, however authentic, inspiring, and supportive, can also just feed your insatiable yearning for information and for thinking. Any good dharma book could be read and studied over and over again to great benefit, only a page or two, or a chapter or two at a time, followed by reflection and sincere attempts to put what you have read into practice. That might take a lifetime.

So quantity is not the issue and the abundance itself can be overwhelming and feed endless doing. In the end, you will have to chart your own course, find your own way, and take readings (i.e., be mindful) from time to time to check and see if the path you are following—the teachers you are finding and the community you are practicing with, if you have found one—feels intuitively healthy and appropriate to your situation and to your aspirations. If not, I suggest you look for other teachers, other resources, another path up the very same mountain.

As you might have gathered from the stories I tell about my Zen teacher Soen Sa Nim (see Books 1 and 4) and about MBSR throughout, it is extremely important to find other like-minded people with whom you can study and practice, and with whom you can talk about your practice. Even one good dharma friend can be a tremendous support to your practice, and being a relationship, its benefits are usually reciprocal...in other words, you wind up supporting each other, and helping yourselves illuminate different aspects of practice just by having conversations about it. You may not even know a lot of the time that it is feeding your practice, but it is.

Forty-five or fifty years ago, you would have been hard-pressed to find a meditation group in even the big cities. Nowadays, they are everywhere. And we can readily find them online. There are vipassana sitting groups and networks around the country and around the world. There are Zen practice groups and Tibetan practice groups. And there are an abundance of meditation centers that offer residential mindfulness retreats of varying lengths, from weekends to several weeks to several months, which you can attend if you care to, where the teachings are superb, offered in English by teachers who have dedicated their lives to the dharma, and to which people come from all over the world. And it is now all at your fingertips.

There are also many hundreds of MBSR programs and CFM-certified teachers in hospitals, clinics, and communities around the country and around the world, where feelings of sangha and community develop spontaneously in the classes, usually in very short order. This expression of sangha winds up being a tremendous support for those who are just getting launched into a mindfulness practice, or who are committing to at least seeing how it would feel over an eight-week period of time, as well as for those who are returning for a "tune-up" and to deepen their practice.

Websites that will take you to such resources for ongoing or periodic support for your practice are also listed at the back of this and the other books in the series.

And then there are the teachers. It can be extremely valuable and instructive to check out different mindfulness teachers and listen carefully to their dharma. With the best of them, the most authentic, you can benefit not just from what they say, but from observing how they carry themselves, from how they are, at least to the degree that they allow themselves to be seen as they actually are. Nobody is perfect, so how they deal or don't deal with their own habits of inattentiveness and greed and aversion when such arise can be very revealing. For practice is not about putting on airs or pretending that one has gotten somewhere, or is blameless or faultless or beyond ordinary feeling states or, for that matter, beyond making mistakes. It is about being real, being authentic, not clinging to anything or recognizing and admitting when one is, and above all, being committed to not wittingly or unwittingly causing harm, and to acting ethically, with integrity and honesty, and warm-heartedness, as best one can.

You can learn a lot by watching how different teachers present the one dharma and embody it in their own lives. Everybody does it differently, and there is no one best or even right way to live mindfully and heartfully in alignment with wisdom. By watching different teachers, you will come to see that you cannot possibly be true to yourself and your own path by merely imitating or revering them, although some of that may happen in the early stages of practice and is not in itself a bad thing. But ultimately, if they are good teachers, they will not encourage a dependency on them. Rather, they will urge you to find your own way, to come to your own understanding through ongoing practice, and to letting life be the teacher, even as you continue to work with them or with other teachers. The Buddha himself stressed that in his dying words, which are purported to be, speaking to his Sangha: "Be a lamp unto yourselves."

And ultimately, you will find that if life is the real teacher, then everybody in your life becomes your teacher, and every moment and occurrence is an opportunity for practice and for seeing beneath the surface appearance of things, and behind your own tendencies to react and contract and close down emotionally, especially when things don't go "your way," and equally so, when they seem to; also in your tendency to think at times that you're a somebody, or in your attempts to strive in some moments to become one or pretend that you are; or in those moments when you know you are a nobody, or your fears arise that you are becoming one, or your ambition makes that its own object of spiritual status and accomplishment.

In all those and many more ways, your most powerful mindfulness teachers may turn out to be your spouse or partner, your children, your parents, other family members, your friends, your colleagues, total strangers, the meter maid giving you a parking ticket, people who actively dislike you, anyone. And of course, the same is true for everything that happens to you. Recall that we said in the previous chapter that, given the appropriate motivation, there are no obstacles to practice, only the appearance of obstacles. Everything supports wakefulness if you are willing to let yourself be awakened by coming to your senses both literally and metaphorically. Everything. But it requires a brave heart, and a mind that sees the folly in clinging...to anything at all, while at the same time, standing in your unique being, with integrity.

When all is said and done, it is always life that is the supreme teacher and the curriculum and the practice. Yet we can benefit enormously from all those people, past, present, and future, who offer us their love and their wisdom and their insights in all the various forms in which they come to us as teachers. They become true blessings in our lives, true gifts to us.

And so in the end, it finally comes full circle, back to your own personal interest in awareness and liberation, to your motivation, your aspiration, your willingness to use whatever arises as opportunities for deepening your commitment to being fully awake, and so, fully alive, no matter what is happening. And these opportunities are not merely for yourself anymore, although that is a perfectly valid place to begin. They are actually nodes in the larger web of interconnectedness, and of life expressing itself through you in the form of perhaps wiser and more compassionate action, not as an ideal or as an idealization of practice, but as a commonsensical way of minimizing suffering and harm in the world, your own and others', and maximizing well-being, kindness, and clarity.

When you commit in such a way, not only can all the above resources become indispensable supports in your practice, there is a way in which, as we will see in *The Healing Power of Mindfulness*, the entire universe "rotates" into alignment with your new view and intentionality. But it is waiting for you to make your move.

As Goethe put it:

Until one is committed, there is always hesitancy, the chance to draw back, always ineffectiveness. Concerning all acts of initiative and creation, there is one elementary truth, the ignorance of which kills countless ideas and splendid plans: the moment one definitely commits oneself, then Providence moves too. All sorts of things occur to help that would never otherwise have occurred. A whole stream of events issues from the decision, raising to one's favor all manner of unforeseen accidents and meetings and material assistance which no man could have dreamed would come his way. Whatever you can do or dream you can, begin it. Boldness has genius, power, and magic in it.

ACKNOWLEDGMENTS

Since the origins of these four volumes go back a long way, there are a number of people to whom I wish to express my gratitude and indebtedness for their many contributions at various stages of the writing and publishing of these books.

For the initial volume, published in 2005, I would like to thank my dharma brother, Larry Rosenberg of the Cambridge Insight Meditation Center, as well as Larry Horwitz, and my father-in-law, the late Howard Zinn, for reading the entire manuscript back in the day and sharing their keen and creative insights with me. My thanks as well to Alan Wallace, Arthur Zajonc, Doug Tanner, and Richard Davidson and to Will Kabat-Zinn and Myla Kabat-Zinn for reading portions of the manuscript and giving me their wise council and feedback. I also thank the original publisher, Bob Miller, and the original editor, Will Schwalbe, now both at Flatiron Books, for their support and friendship, then and now.

Deep and special appreciation, gratitude, and indebtedness to my editor of the first volume, Michelle Howry, executive editor at Hachette Books, who helped midwife the form of the entire series; to Lauren Hummel for her key contributions to making sure all went well, and skillfully keeping all of the moving parts of this project on track; and to the entire Hachette team that worked so cooperatively and effectively on this series. Also, deep appreciation to Mauro DiPreta, vice president and publisher of Hachette

Books, who stepped in to edit the last three volumes when Michelle moved on.

While I have received support, encouragement, and advice from many, of course any inaccuracies or shortcomings in the text are entirely my own.

I wish to express enduring gratitude and respect to all my teaching colleagues, past and present in the Stress Reduction Clinic and the Center for Mindfulness and, more recently, also to those teachers and researchers who are part of the CFM's global network of affiliate institutions. All have literally and metaphorically dedicated their lives and their passion to this work. At the time of the original book, those who had taught MBSR in the Stress Reduction Clinic for varying periods of time from 1979 to 2005 were Saki Santorelli, Melissa Blacker, Florence Meleo-Meyer, Elana Rosenbaum, Ferris Buck Urbanowski, Pamela Erdmann, Fernando de Torrijos, James Carmody, Danielle Levi Alvares, George Mumford, Diana Kamila, Peggy Roggenbuck-Gillespie, Debbie Beck, Zayda Vallejo, Barbara Stone, Trudy Goodman, Meg Chang, Larry Rosenberg, Kasey Carmichael, Franz Moekel, the late Ulli Kesper-Grossman, Maddy Klein, Ann Soulet, Joseph Koppel, the late Karen Ryder, Anna Klegon, Larry Pelz, Adi Bemak, Paul Galvin, and David Spound.

In 2018, my admiration and gratitude go to the current teachers in the Center for Mindfulness and its affiliate programs: Florence Meleo-Meyers, Lynn Koerbel, Elana Rosenbaum, Carolyn West, Bob Stahl, Meg Chang, Zayda Vallejo, Brenda Fingold, Dianne Horgan, Judson Brewer, Margaret Fletcher, Patti Holland, Rebecca Eldridge, Ted Meissner, Anne Twohig, Ana Arrabe, Beth Mulligan, Bonita Jones, Carola Garcia, Gustavo Diex, Beatriz Rodriguez, Melissa Tefft, Janet Solyntjes, Rob Smith, Jacob Piet, Claude Maskens, Charlotte Borch-Jacobsen, Christiane Wolf,

Kate Mitcheom, Bob Linscott, Laurence Magro, Jim Colosi, Julie Nason, Lone Overby Fjorback, Dawn MacDonald, Leslie Smith Frank, Ruth Folchman, Colleen Camenisch, Robin Boudette, Eowyn Ahlstrom, Erin Woo, Franco Cuccio, Geneviève Hamelet, Gwenola Herbette, and Ruth Whitall. Florence Meleo-Meyer and Lynn Koerbel have been outstanding leaders and nurturers of the global network of MBSR teachers at the CFM.

Profound appreciation to all those who contributed so critically in so many different ways to the administration of the MBSR Clinic and the Center for Mindfulness in Medicine, Health Care, and Society and to their various research and clinical endeavors from the very beginning: Norma Rosiello, Kathy Brady, Brian Tucker, Anne Skillings, Tim Light, Jean Baril, Leslie Lynch, Carol Lewis, Leigh Emery, Rafaela Morales, Roberta Lewis, Jen Gigliotti, Sylvia Ciario, Betty Flodin, Diane Spinney, Carol Hester, Carol Mento, Olivia Hobletzell, the late Narina Hendry, Marlene Samuelson, Janet Parks, Michael Bratt, Marc Cohen, and Ellen Wingard; and in the current era, building on a robust platform developed under the leadership of Saki Santorelli over seventeen years, I extend my gratitude to the current leadership of Judson Brewer, Dianne Horgan, Florence Meleo-Meyer, and Lynn Koerbel, with amazing support from Jean Baril, Jacqueline Clark, Tony Maciag, Ted Meissner, Jessica Novia, Maureen Titus, Beverly Walton, Ashley Gladden, Lynne Littizzio, Nicole Rocijewicz, and Jean Welker. And a deep bow to Judson Brewer, MD, PhD, who became, in 2017, the founding director of the Division of Mindfulness in the Department of Medicine at the University of Massachusetts Medical School—the first division of mindfulness in a medical school in the world, and very much a sign of the times and of the promise of things to come.

On the research side of the CFM in 2018, robust appreciation for the breadth and depth of your work and contributions: Judson

Brewer, Remko van Lutterveld, Prasanta Pal, Michael Datko, Andrea Ruf, Susan Druker, Ariel Beccia, Alexandra Roy, Hanif Benoit, Danny Theisen, and Carolyn Neal.

Finally, I would also like to express my gratitude and respect for the thousands of people everywhere around the world who work in or are researching mindfulness-based approaches in medicine, psychiatry, psychology, health care, education, the law, social justice, refugee healing in the face of trauma and sometimes genocide (as in South Darfur), childbirth and parenting, the workplace, government, prisons, and other facets of society, and who take care to honor the dharma in its universal depth and beauty in doing so. You know who you are, whether you are named here or not! And if you are not, it is only due to my own shortcomings and the limits of space. I want to explicitly honor the work of Paula Andrea Ramirez Diazgranados in Columbia and South Darfur; Hui Qi Tong in the U.S. and China; Kevin Fong, Roy Te Chung Chen, Tzungkuen Wen, Helen Ma, Jin Mei Hu, and Shih Shih Ming in China, Taiwan, and Hong Kong; Heyoung Ahn in Korea; Junko Bickel and Teruro Shiina in Japan; Leena Pennenen in Finland; Simon Whitesman and Linda Kantor in South Africa; Claude Maskens, Gwénola Herbette, Edel Max, Caroline Lesire, and Ilios Kotsou in Belgium; Jean-Gérard Bloch, Geneviève Hamelet, Marie-Ange Pratili, and Charlotte Borch-Jacobsen in France; Katherine Bonus, Trish Magyari, Erica Sibinga, David Kearney, Kurt Hoelting, Carolyn McManus, Mike Brumage, Maureen Strafford, Amy Gross, Rhonda Magee, George Mumford, Carl Fulwiler, Maria Kluge, Mick Krasner, Trish Luck, Bernice Todres, Ron Epstein, and Representative Tim Ryan in the U.S.: Paul Grossman, Maria Kluge, Sylvia Wiesman-Fiscalini, Linda Hehrhaupt, and Petra Meibert in Germany; Joke Hellemans, Johan Tinge, and Anna Speckens in Holland; Beatrice Heller and Regula Saner in

Switzerland; Rebecca Crane, Willem Kuyken, John Teasdale, Mark Williams, Chris Cullen, Richard Burnett, Jamie Bristow, Trish Bartley, Stewart Mercer, Chris Ruane, Richard Layard, Guiaume Hung, and Ahn Nguyen in the UK; Zindel Segal and Norm Farb in Canada; Gabor Fasekas in Hungary; Macchi dela Vega in Argentina; Johan Bergstad, Anita Olsson, Angeli Holmstedt; Ola Schenström, and Camilla Sköld in Sweden; Andries Kroese in Norway; Jakob Piet and Lone Overby Fjorback in Denmark; and Franco Cuccio in Italy. May your work continue to reach those who are most in need of it, touching, clarifying, and nurturing what is deepest and best in us all, and thus contributing, in ways little and big to the healing and transformation that humanity so sorely longs for and aspires to.

RELATED READINGS

Mindfulness Meditation

Amero, B. *Small Boat, Great Mountain: Theravadan Reflections on the Great Natural Perfection*, Abhayagiri Monastic Foundation, Redwood Valley, CA, 2003.

Analayo, B. *Early Buddhist Meditation Studies*, Barre Center for Buddhist Studies, Barre, MA, 2017.

Analayo, B. *Mindfully Facing Disease and Death: Compassionate Advice from Early Buddhist Texts*, Windhorse, Cambridge, UK, 2016.

Analayo, B. *Satipatthana: The Direct Path to Realization*, Windhorse, Cambridge, UK, 2008.

Armstrong, G. *Emptiness: A Practical Guide for Meditators I*, Wisdom, Somerville, MA, 2017.

Beck, C. *Nothing Special: Living Zen*, HarperCollins, San Francisco, 1993.

Buswell, R. B., Jr. *Tracing Back the Radiance: Chinul's Korean Way of Zen*, Kuroda Institute, U of Hawaii Press, Honolulu, 1991.

Goldstein, J. *Mindfulness: A Practical Guide to Awakening*, Sounds True, Boulder, CO, 2013.

Goldstein, J. *One Dharma: The Emerging Western Buddhism*, HarperCollins, San Francisco, 2002.

Goldstein, J. and Kornfield, J. *Seeking the Heart of Wisdom: The Path of Insight Meditation*, Shambhala, Boston, 1987.

Gunaratana, H. *Mindfulness in Plain English*, Wisdom, Boston, 1996.

Hanh, T. N. *The Heart of the Buddha's Teachings*, Broadway, New York, 1998.

Hanh, T. N. *How to Love*, Parallax Press, Berkeley, 2015

Hanh, T. N. *How to Sit*, Parallax Press, Berkeley, 2014.

Hanh, T. N. *The Miracle of Mindfulness*, Beacon, Boston, 1976.

Kapleau, P. *The Three Pillars of Zen: Teaching, Practice, and Enlightenment*, Random House, New York, 1965, 2000.

Krishnamurti, J. *This Light in Oneself: True Meditation*, Shambhala, Boston, 1999.

Levine, S. *A Gradual Awakening*, Anchor/Doubleday, Garden City, NY, 1979.

Ricard, R. *Happiness*. Little Brown, New York, 2007.

Ricard, R. *Why Meditate?*, Hay House, New York, 2010.

Rinpoche, M. *The Joy of Wisdom*, Harmony Books, New York, 2010.

Rosenberg, L. *Breath by Breath: The Liberating Practice of Insight Meditation*, Shambhala, Boston, 1998.

Rosenberg, L. *Living in the Light of Death: On the Art of Being Truly Alive*, Shambhala, Boston, 2000.

Rosenberg, L. *Three Steps to Awakening: A Practice for Bringing Mindfulness to Life*, Shambhala, Boston, 2013.

Salzberg, S. *Lovingkindness*, Shambhala, Boston, 1995.

Salzberg, S. *Real Love: The Art of Mindful Connection*, Flatiron Books, New York, 2017.

Sheng-Yen, C. *Hoofprints of the Ox: Principles of the Chan Buddhist Path*, Oxford University Press, New York, 2001.

Soeng, M. *The Heart of the Universe: Exploring the Heart Sutra*. Wisdom, Somerville, MA, 2010.

Soeng, M. *Trust in Mind: The Rebellion of Chinese Zen*. Wisdom, Somerville, MA, 2004.

Sumedo, A. *The Mind and the Way: Buddhist Reflections on Life*, Wisdom, Boston, 1995.

Suzuki, S. *Zen Mind, Beginner's Mind*, Weatherhill, New York, 1970.

Thera, N. *The Heart of Buddhist Meditation: The Buddha's Way of Mindfulness*, Red Wheel/Weiser, San Francisco, 1962, 2014.

Treleaven, D. *Trauma-Sensitive Mindfulness: Practices for Safe and Transformative Healing*, W.W. Norton, New York, 2018.

Tulku Urgyen. *Rainbow Painting*, Rangjung Yeshe: Boudhanath, Nepal, 1995.

MBSR

Brandsma, R. *The Mindfulness Teaching Guide: Essential Skills and Competencies for Teaching Mindfulness-Based Interventions*, New Harbinger, Oakland, CA, 2017.

Kabat-Zinn, J. *Full Catastrophe Living: Using the Wisdom of Your Body and Mind to Face Stress, Pain, and Illness*, revised and updated edition, Random House, New York, 2013.

Lehrhaupt, L. and Meibert, P. *Mindfulness-Based Stress Reduction: The MBSR Program for Enhancing Health and Vitality*, New World Library, Novato, CA, 2017.

Mulligan, B. A. *The Dharma of Modern Mindfulness: Discovering the Buddhist Teachings at the Heart of Mindfulness-Based Stress Reduction*, New Harbinger, Oakland, CA, 2017.

Rosenbaum, E. *The Heart of Mindfulness-Based Stress Reduction: An MBSR Guide for Clinicians and Clients*, Pesi Publishing, Eau Claire, WI, 2017.

Santorelli, S. *Heal Thy Self: Lessons on Mindfulness in Medicine*, Bell Tower, New York, 1999.

Stahl, B. and Goldstein, E. *A Mindfulness-Based Stress Reduction Workbook*, New Harbinger, Oakland, CA, 2010.

Stahl, B., Meleo-Meyer, F., and Koerbel, L. *A Mindfulness-Based Stress Reduction Workbook for Anxiety*, New Harbinger, Oakland, CA, 2014.

Other Applications of Mindfulness

Bardacke, N. *Mindful Birthing: Training the Mind, Body, and Heart for Childbirth and Beyond*, HarperCollins, New York, 2012.

Bartley, T. *Mindfulness: A Kindly Approach to Cancer*, Wiley-Blackwell, West Sussex, UK, 2016.

Bartley, T. *Mindfulness-Based Cognitive Therapy for Cancer*, Wiley-Blackwell, West Sussex, UK, 2012.

Bays, J. C. *Mindful Eating: A Guide to Rediscovering a Healthy and Joyful Relationship with Food*, Shambhala, Boston, 2009, 2017.

Bays, J. C. *Mindfulness on the Go: Simple Meditation Practices You Can Do Anywhere*, Shambhala, Boston, 2014.

Biegel, G. *The Stress-Reduction Workbook for Teens: Mindfulness Skills to Help You Deal with Stress*, New Harbinger, Oakland, CA, 2017.

Brantley, J. *Calming Your Anxious Mind: How Mindfulness and Compassion Can Free You from Anxiety, Fear, and Panic*, New Harbinger, Oakland, CA, 2003.

Brewer, Judson. *The Craving Mind: From Cigarettes to Smartphones to Love— Why We Get Hooked and How We Can Break Bad Habits*, Yale University Press, New Haven, 2017

Brown, K. W., Creswell, J. D., and Ryan, R. M. (eds). *Handbook of Mindfulness: Theory, Research, and Practice*, Guilford, New York, 2015.

Carlson, L. and Speca, M. *Mindfulness-Based Cancer Recovery: A Step-by-Step MBSR Approach to Help You Cope with Treatment and Reclaim Your Life*, New Harbinger, Oakland, CA, 2010.

Cullen, M. and Pons, G. B. *The Mindfulness-Based Emotional Balance Workbook: An Eight-Week Program for Improved Emotion Regulation and Resilience*, New Harbinger, Oakland, CA, 2015.

Epstein, M. *Thoughts Without a Thinker*, Basic Books, New York, 1995.

Epstein, R. *Attending: Medicine, Mindfulness, and Humanity*, Scribner, New York, 2017.

Germer, C. *The Mindful Path to Self-Compassion*, Guilford, New York, 2009.

Goleman, D. *Destructive Emotions: How We Can Heal Them*, Bantam, NY, 2003.

Goleman, G, and Davidson, R. J. *Altered Traits: Science Reveals How Meditation Changes Your Mind, Brain, and Body*, Avery/Random House, New York, 2017.

Gunaratana, B. H. *Mindfulness in Plain English*, Wisdom, Somerville, MA, 2002.

Harris, N. B. *The Deepest Well: Healing the Long-term Effects of Childhood Adversity*, Houghton Mifflin Harcout, Boston, 2018.

Jennings, P. *Mindfulness for Teachers: Simple Skills for Peace and Productivity in the Classroom*, W.W. Norton, New York, 2015.

Jones, A. *Beyond Vision: Going Blind, Inner Seeing, and the Nature of the Self*, McGill-Queen's University Press, Montreal, 2018.

Kaiser-Greenland, S. *Mindful Games: Sharing Mindfulness and Games with Children, Teen, and Families*, Shambhala, Boulder, CO, 2016.

Kaiser-Greenland, S. *The Mindful Child*, Free Press, New York, 2010.

Kaufman, K. A., Glass, C. R., and Pineau, T. R. *Mindful Sport Performance Enhancement: Mental Training for Athletes and Coaches*, American Psychological Association (APA), Washington, DC, 2018.

McCown, D., Reibel, D., and Micozzi, M. S. (eds.). *Resources for Teaching Mindfulness: An International Handbook*, Springer, New York, 2016.

McCown, D., Reibel, D., and Micozzi, M. S. (eds.). *Teaching Mindfulness: A Practical Guide for Clinicians and Educators*, Springer, New York, 2010.

McManus, C.A. *Group Wellness Programs for Chronic Pain and Disease Management*, Butterworth-Heinemann, St. Louis, MO, 2003.

Mumford, G. *The Mindful Athlete: Secrets to Pure Performance*, Parallax Press, Berkeley, 2015.

Penman, D. *The Art of Breathing*, Conari, Newburyport, MA, 2018.

Rechtschaffen, D. *The Mindful Education Workbook: Lessons for Teaching Mindfulness to Students*, W.W. Norton, New York, 2016.

Rechtschaffen, D. *The Way of Mindful Education: Cultivating Wellbeing in Teachers and Students*, W.W. Norton, New York, 2014.

Rosenbaum, E. *Being Well (Even When You Are Sick): Mindfulness Practices for People with Cancer and Other Serious Illnesses*, Shambala, Boston, 2012.

Rosenbaum, E. *Here for Now: Living Well with Cancer Through Mindfulness*, Satya House, Hardwick, MA, 2005.

Segal, Z. V., Williams, J. M. G., and Teasdale, J. D. *Mindfulness-Based Cognitive Therapy for Depression: A New Approach to Preventing Relapse*, second edition, Guilford, New York, 2013.

Teasdale, J. D., Williams, M., and Segal, Z. V. *The Mindful Way Workbook: An Eight-Week Program to Free Yourself from Depression and Emotional Distress*, Guilford, New York, 2014.

Tolle, E. *The Power of Now*, New World Library, Novato, CA, 1999.

Wallace, B.A. *Tibetan Buddhism from the Ground Up*, Wisdom, Somerville, MA, 1993.

Williams, A. K., Owens, R., and Syedullah, J. *Radical Dharma: Talking Race, Love, and Liberation*, North Atlantic Books, Berkeley, 2016.

Williams, J. M. G., Teasdale, J. D., Segal, Z. V., and Kabat-Zinn, J. *The Mindful Way Through Depression: Freeing Yourself from Chronic Unhappiness*, Guilford, New York, 2007.

Williams, M. and Penman, D. *Mindfulness: An Eight-Week Plan for Finding Peace in a Frantic World*, Rodale, New York, 2012.

Yang, L. *Awakening Together: The Spiritual Practice of Inclusivity and Community*, Wisdom, Somerville, MA, 2017.

Healing

Doidge, N. *The Brain's Way of Healing: Remarkable Discoveries and Recoveries from the Frontiers of Neuroplasticity*, Penguin Random House, New York, 2016.

Goleman, D. *Healing Emotions: Conversations with the Dalai Lama on Mindfulness, Emotions, and Health*, Shambhala, Boston, 1997.

Moyers, B. *Healing and the Mind*, Doubleday, New York, 1993.

Ornish, D. *Love and Survival: The Scientific Basis for the Healing Power of Intimacy*, HaperCollins, New York, 1998.

Remen, R. *Kitchen Table Wisdom: Stories that Heal*, Riverhead, New York, 1997.

Siegel, D. *The Mindful Brain: Reflection and Attunement in the Cultivation of Wellbeing*, W.W. Norton, New York, 2007.

Simmons, P. *Learning to Fall: The Blessings of an Imperfect Life*, Bantam, New York, 2002.

Tarrant, J. *The Light Inside the Dark: Zen, Soul, and the Spiritual Life*, HarperCollins, New York, 1998.

Tenzin Gyatso (the 14th Dalai Lama). *The Compassionate Life*, Wisdom, Boston, 2003.

Van der Kolk, B. *The Body Keeps the Score: Brain, Mind, and Body in the Healing of Trauma*, Penguin Random House, New York, 2014.

Poetry

Eliot, T. S. *Four Quartets*, Harcourt Brace, New York, 1943, 1977.

Lao-Tzu, *Tao Te Ching*, (Stephen Mitchell, transl.), HarperCollins, New York, 1988.

Mitchell, S. *The Enlightened Heart*, Harper & Row, New York, 1989.

Oliver, M. *New and Selected Poems*, Beacon, Boston, 1992.

Tanahashi, K. and Leavitt, P. *The Complete Cold Mountain: Poems of the Legendary Hermit, Hanshan*, Shambhala, Boulder, CO, 2018.

Whyte, D. *The Heart Aroused: Poetry and the Preservation of the Soul in Corporate America*, Doubleday, New York, 1994.

Other Books of Interest, Some Mentioned in the Text

Abram, D. *The Spell of the Sensuous*, Vintage, New York, 1996.

Ackerman, D. *A Natural History of the Senses*, Vintage, New York, 1990.

Blackburn, E. and Epel, E. *The Telomere Effect: A Revolutionary Approach to Living Younger, Healthier, Longer*, Grand Central Publishing, New York, 2017.

Bohm, D. *Wholeness and the Implicate Order*, Routledge and Kegan Paul, London, 1980.

Bryson, B. *A Short History of Nearly Everything*, Broadway, New York, 2003.

Davidson, R. J., and Begley, S. *The Emotional Life of Your Brain*, Hudson St. Press, New York, 2012.

Glassman, B. *Bearing Witness: A Zen Master's Lessons in Making Peace*, Bell Tower, New York, 1998.

Greene, B. *The Elegant Universe*, Norton, New York, 1999.

Harris, Y. N. *Sapiens: A Brief History of Humankind*, HarperCollins, New York, 2015.

Hillman, J. *The Soul's Code: In Search of Character and Calling*, Random House, New York, 1996.

Karr-Morse, R. and Wiley, M. S. *Ghosts from the Nursery: Tracing the Roots of Violence*, Atlantic Monthly Press, New York, 1997.

Katie, B. and Mitchell, S. *A Mind at Home with Itself*, HarperCollins, New York, 2017.

Kazanjian, V. H., and Laurence, P. L. (eds.). *Education as Transformation*, Peter Lang, New York, 2000.

Kurzweil, R. *The Age of Spiritual Machines*, Viking, New York, 1999.

Luke, H. *Old Age: Journey into Simplicity*, Parabola, New York, 1987.

Montague, A. *Touching: The Human Significance of the Skin*, Harper & Row, New York, 1978.

Palmer, P. *The Courage to Teach: Exploring the Inner Landscape of a Teacher's Life*, Jossey-Bass, San Francisco, 1998.

Pinker, S. *The Better Angels of Our Nature: Why Violence Has Declined*, Penguin Random House, New York, 2012.

Pinker, S. *Enlightenment Now: The Case for Reason, Science, Humanism, and Progress*, Penguin Random House, New York, 2018.

Pinker, S. *How the Mind Works*, W.W. Norton, New York, 1997.

Ravel, J.-F. and Ricard, M. *The Monk and the Philosopher: A Father and Son Discuss the Meaning of Life*, Schocken, New York, 1998.

Ricard, M. *Altruism: The Power of Compassion to Change Yourself and the World*, Little Brown, New York, 2013.

Ryan, T. *A Mindful Nation: How a Simple Practice Can Help Us Reduce Stress, Improve Performance, and Recapture the American Spirit*, Hay House, New York, 2012.

Sachs, J. D. *The Price of Civilization: Reawakening American Virtue and Prosperity*, Random House, New York, 2011.

Sachs, O. *The Man Who Mistook His Wife for a Hat*, Touchstone, New York, 1970.

Sachs, O. *The River of Consciousness*, Knopf, New York, 2017.

Sapolsky, R. *Behave: The Biology of Humans at Our Best and Worst*, Penguin Random House, New York, 2017.

Schwartz, J. M. and Begley, S. *The Mind and the Brain: Neuroplasticity and the Power of Mental Force*, HarperCollins, New York, 2002.

Singh, S. *Fermat's Enigma*, Anchor, New York, 1997.

Tanahashi, K. *The Heart Sutra: A Comprehensive Guide to the Classic of Mahayana Buddhism*, Shambhala, Boulder, CO, 2016.

Tegmark, M. *Life 3.0: Being Human in the Age of Artificial Intelligence*, Knopf, New York, 2017.

Tegmark, M. *The Mathematical Universe: My Quest for the Ultimate Nature of Reality*, Random House, New York, 2014.

Turkle, S. *Alone Together: Why We Expect More from Technology and Less from Each Other*, Basic Books, New York, 2011.

Turkle, S. *Reclaiming Conversation: The Power of Talk in a Digital Age*, Penguin Random House, New York, 2015.

Varela, F. J., Thompson, E., and Rosch, E. *The Embodied Mind: Cognitive Science and Human Experience*, revised edition, MIT Press, Cambridge, MA, 2016.

Wright, R. *Why Buddhism Is True: The Science and Philosophy of Meditation and Enlightenment*, Simon & Schuster, New York, 2017.

Websites

www.umassmed.edu/cfm	Website of the Center for Mindfulness, UMass Medical School
www.mindandlife.org	Website of the Mind and Life Institute
www.dharma.org	Vipassana retreat centers and schedules

INDEX

ABOUT THE AUTHOR

Jon Kabat-Zinn, Ph.D., is the founder of MBSR (mindfulness-based stress reduction) and the Stress Reduction Clinic (1979) and of the Center for Mindfulness in Medicine, Health Care, and Society (1995) at the University of Massachusetts Medical School. He is also professor of Medicine emeritus. He leads workshops and retreats on mindfulness for health professionals, the tech and business communities, and for lay audiences worldwide. He is a strong proponent of social justice and economic justice. He is the author or coauthor of ten books, including the bestselling *Wherever You Go, There You Are* and *Full Catastrophe Living*. With his wife Myla Kabat-Zinn, he published a book on mindful parenting, *Everyday Blessings*. He has been featured in numerous documentaries for television around the world, including the PBS Special *Healing and the Mind* with Bill Moyers, *Oprah*, and CBS's *60 Minutes* with Anderson Cooper. He lives in Massachusetts. His work has contributed to a growing movement of mindfulness into mainstream institutions such as medicine, psychology, health care, neuroscience, schools, higher education, business, social justice, criminal justice, prisons, the law, technology, government, and professional sports. Hospitals and medical centers around the world now offer clinical programs based on training in mindfulness and MBSR.

Continue the journey and get the full set of
Jon Kabat-Zinn's four small-but-mighty guides to
mindfulness and meditation, as well as his
bestselling classic *Wherever You Go, There You Are.*

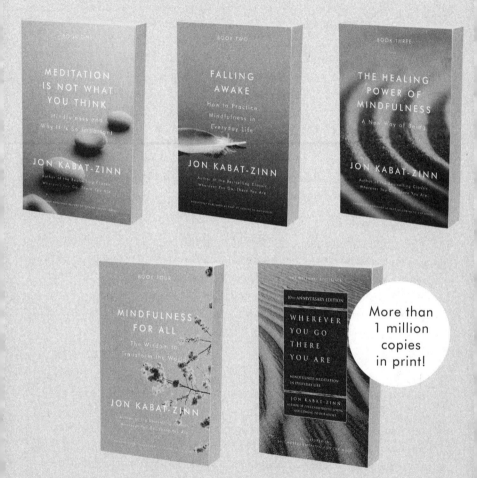

JON KABAT-ZINN, PhD, is the founder of Mindfulness-Based
Stress Reduction (MBSR) and of the Center for Mindfulness in Medicine,
Health Care and Society at the University of Massachusetts, where he
is Professor of Medicine emeritus. He is the author of numerous bestselling books about mindfulness and meditation. For more information,
visit www.jonkabat-zinn.com.

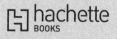
hachette
BOOKS

Guided Mindfulness Meditation Practices with Jon Kabat-Zinn

**Obtainable as apps, downloads, or CDs
(see below for links)**

Series 1

These guided meditations (the body scan and sitting meditation) and guided mindful yoga practices 1 and 2 form the foundational practices of MBSR and are used in MBSR programs around the world. These practices and their use are described in detail in *Full Catastrophe Living*. Each meditation is 45 minutes in length.

Series 2

These guided meditations are designed for people who want a range of shorter guided meditations to help them develop and/or expand and deepen a personal meditation practice based on mindfulness. The series includes the mountain and lake meditations (each 20 minutes) as well as a range of other 10-minute, 20-minute, and 30-minute sitting and lying down practices. This series was originally developed to accompany *Wherever You Go, There You Are*.

Series 3

These guided meditations are designed to accompany this book and the other three volumes based on *Coming to Our Senses*. Series 3 includes guided meditations on the breath and body sensations (breathscape and bodyscape), on sounds (soundscape), thoughts and emotions (mindscape), choiceless awareness (nowscape), and lovingkindness (heartscape), as well as instructions for lying down meditation (corpse pose/dying before you die), mindful walking, and cultivating mindfulness in everyday life (lifescape).

For iPhone and Android apps: www.mindfulnessapps.com

For digital downloads: www.betterlisten.com/pages/jonkabatzinnseries123

For CD sets: www.soundstrue.com/jon-kabat-zinn